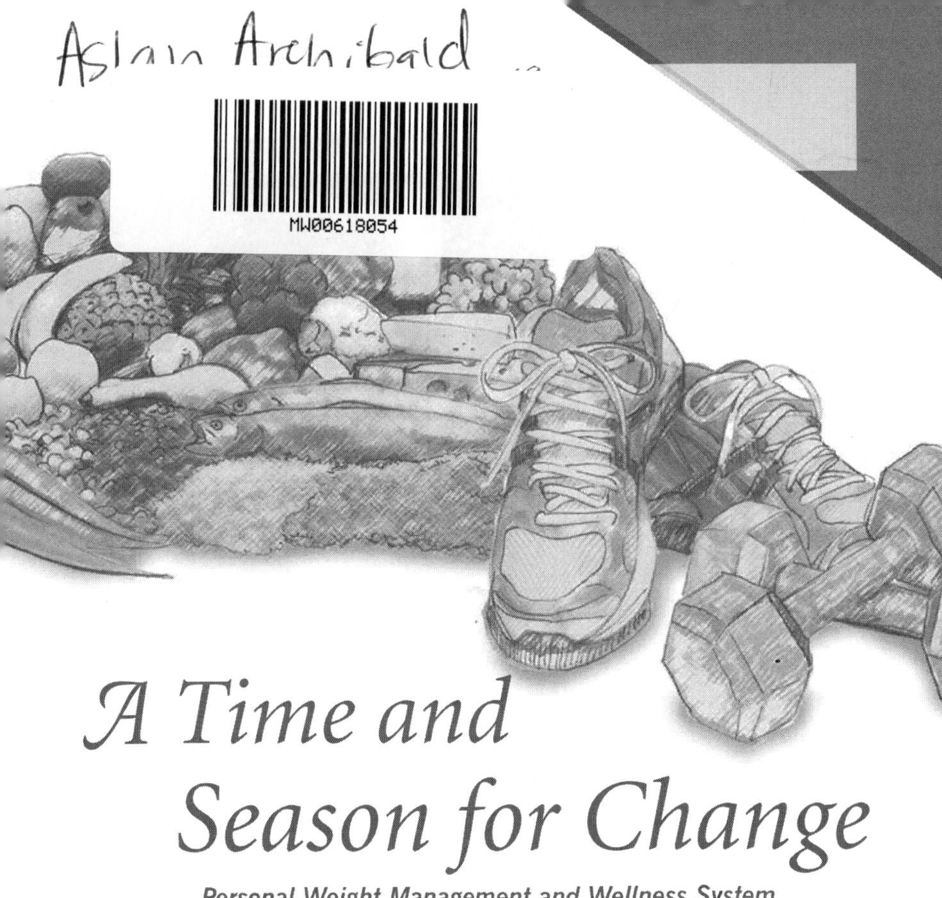

# *A Time and Season for Change*

***Personal Weight Management and Wellness System***

About the Author:

Lynn R. Perkes MS, ATC, is a faculty member at Brigham Young University-Idaho in the Department of Health, Recreation and Human Performance. His primary classes include Health and Fitness Appraisal and Prescription and Introduction to Kinesiology and Biomechanics. Previously he has worked in industry developing and implementing health, fitness, wellness and weight management programs.

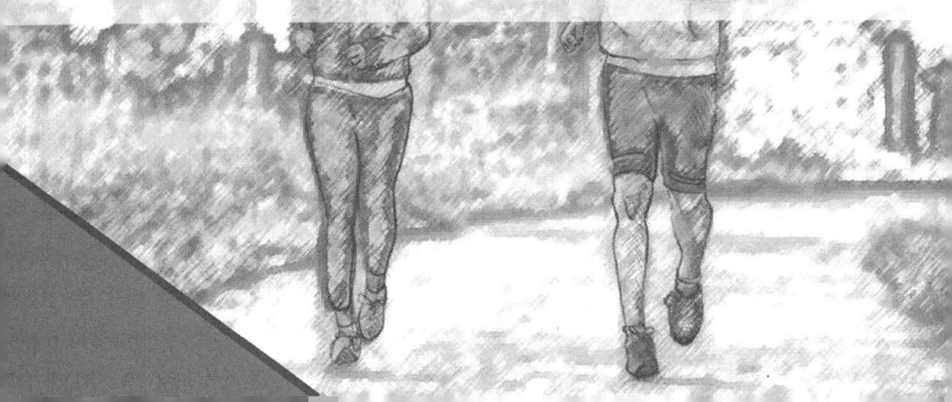

A Time and Season for Change:
Personal Weight Management and Wellness System

Lynn Robert Perkes, MS, ATC


Published by Hidden Valley Publishing
www.hiddenvalleypublishing.com

atimeandseasonforchange@gmail.com

ISBN # 978-0-9897596-1-8

Notice and Disclaimer
The information in this book provides general guidelines for nutrition, fitness and behavioral modification as an educational framework and is not intended to provide medical advice or to substitute for the advice of your physician.

It is recommended that the user of this book consult his or her physician before beginning any nutritional, weight loss, or exercise program.

The publisher specifically disclaims any responsibility for any liability, loss or risk, personal or otherwise, which is incurred as a consequence, directly or indirectly, of the use and application of any of the contents of this book.

## Table of Contents

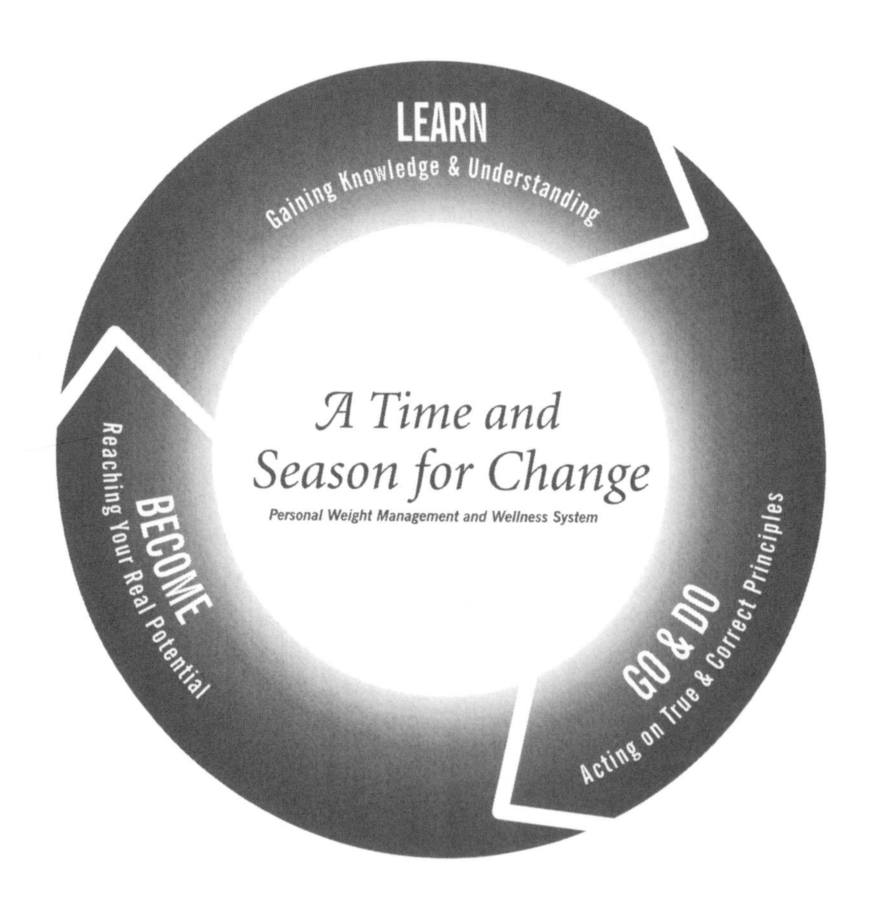
LEARN
Gaining Knowledge & Understanding
GO & DO
Acting on True & Correct Principles
BECOME
Reaching Your Real Potential
A Time and
Season for Change
Personal Weight Management and Wellness System

# Your Personal Weight Management and Wellness System

Welcome to what we hope will be, and what truly should be, a time and season of your life for personal lifestyle change. Change directed toward a leaner and healthier you; more capable of going, doing, and becoming. Most individuals who achieve real and lasting success usually report a significant life event or a moment of intense realization that helped create in themselves an unalterable drive and motivation to do whatever it takes to achieve their long desired goals.

Have you come to this point in your life where you truly want to make meaningful change, to persist – sometimes under challenging conditions – until you achieve your success, and to effectively alter your future for the better? If so, it is vitally important to understand that one of the great privileges and responsibilities we have in this life is the gift of ***agency***, the capacity and freedom to ***act*** for ourselves, and not merely be acted upon. This power for independent ***action***, when guided by true and correct principles, becomes an enabling power to help us more effectively govern our lives; with success, enjoyment, progress and meaningful growth being the fruits of our efforts. If however, our choices and actions are influenced or directed by false and incorrect principles then we are being acted upon; and failure, frustration, and discouragement are often the result. Your lifestyle change and associated benefits will come as a result of your personal commitment and diligence to the application of true and correct principles. Not from gimmicks or fads, but evidence-based concepts and principles that have stood the test of scientific research and have proven results.

The principles, strategies and tools for proper nutrition, fitness, weight management and wellness set forth in this Personal Weight Management and Wellness System are derived from evidence-based data, guidelines and principles from the Dietary Approaches to Stopping Hypertension (DASH) Diet, the Mediterranean Diet, the National Institutes of Health report *Clinical Guidelines on the Identification, Evaluation and Treatment of Overweight and Obesity in Adults*, the National Weight Control Registry, and the American College of Sports Medicine. Collectively they represent a wealth of knowledge and put forth correct principles that have helped those seeking to make change a reality in their lives. When properly practiced they allow us to more effectively govern our lives toward achieving a healthier and leaner body.

We have been blessed with one body, a marvelous and capable body. It is our privilege and responsibility to care for it that it might serve us well in the essence of life; having the capacity to do, to become, to serve, to contribute, and to be there for our family and friends.

The invitation is extended to you to invest in yourself and truly make this your season of change; a time to study, learn, understand and effectively apply (***act upon***) these correct principles and proven strategies in your life toward reaching your real potential. By so doing you are choosing to ***act*** for yourself and you become the governing influence for accomplishment in your own life. Make the decision now to actively pursue and persist until you reach your goals, and make this your time and your season for change. You and those who love you best are certainly worth it. So, let's get started!

# How to Use Your Personal Weight Management and Wellness System

As with any worthy effort we must begin by increasing our knowledge and understanding of the principles and skills that are essential to performing the tasks that lie ahead. This process is an investment in yourself that will not only help you achieve the desired success, but because of your increased abilities will positively impact every aspect of your life, enabling you with greater capacity to live up to your potential.

The following sequential "steps" are designed to engage you in the process of evaluation, goal setting, learning, doing, and ultimately becoming as you ***act*** upon true and correct principles toward meaningful lifestyle change. Take the time to read and study each step, incorporate its teachings and purposes into your behavior and thought processes, and emerge as a new person more capable and qualified to ***act*** for yourself in achieving your goals.

**√ = when completed and then move on to the next step**

❏ **Step 1**: Participate in an exploratory and evaluative process by completing the **Personal Awareness and Readiness for Change Assessment Tool.** This assessment tool is an important preparatory step in your progress toward personal change and becoming. (See page 7)

❏ **Step 2**: As you begin your journey of change and becoming it is strongly recommended that you obtain some baseline **health and fitness measurements**. These measured values can serve as important points from which to set goals, measure progress, and establish rewards for when you accomplish your goals. In the section to record your baseline measurements (See page 11) are a number of different health and fitness assessments in which you may choose to be evaluated. Because this program is used in a variety of settings (personal use, classroom, wellness coaches, personal trainers), there are a variety of tests including body weight, BMI, circumference measurements, blood pressure, blood cholesterol, cardiorespiratory-VO2max, muscular fitness, flexibility, etc. However, depending on your circumstances, available resources, and personal preference, select those assessments you truly want to track overtime and which can serve as benchmarks for evaluation of your progress in those areas most important to you. If desired, seek out individuals and/or facilities that offer the additional tests you desire or simply perform the basic measures yourself, e.g. weight, circumference measurements, etc.

❏ **Step 3**: You obviously have at least one goal as part of your time and season for change efforts – to lose excess body fat. Equally important, we hope that through your efforts you will develop and incorporate a culture of **wellness** into your everyday life – actively engaged in attitudes and behaviors that enhance your quality of life and maximize your personal potential. In the "**Goals and Rewards**" section (See page 13) carefully consider what you truly want to achieve in the areas of body weight, health, fitness, or other wellness category important to you, and record your goals. Review them often as a reminder of what you have determined as priorities in your life. Commit and recommit to do what is needed to accomplish your goals. Work hard (***acting***) to make them a reality, and appropriately reward yourself for your successes as you continue your forward progress toward change and becoming.

❏ **Step 4**: This step is where much of the **learning – gaining knowledge and wisdom of key principles and appropriate processes** must occur in preparation for your journey. As you acquire new knowledge, skills and understanding you are better prepared to ***act*** in making appropriate behavioral changes in a line upon line process. This acquisition of new knowledge and skills can be fun, exciting and motivating. Immerse yourself in the study of these principles and engage in the process with the attitude of an adventure that will in the end, result in an empowered you more capable of doing and becoming. (See page 15)

❑ **Step 5**: This step is where you use evidence-based energy equations to calculate and customize your nutritional plan which will serve as the foundational framework of your weight loss program. Using your own physical dimensions of weight, height, age and gender you will calculate your **Resting Metabolic Rate** (RMR) and your **Activities of Daily Living** (ADL) values. These values, explained in detail in this section, give you the needed information to determine the **Nutritional Plan Calorie Level** (NPCL) you should consume, customized specifically for you, to achieve a **negative energy balance**, causing your body to draw upon its own fat stores for energy metabolism and leads to weight loss. The calculations are simple, the process is fun, and the resulting energy usage information about your body will help in the understanding of how you should eat for health and weight loss according to the uniqueness's of your body and its metabolism. (See page 33)

Also determined from these values will be the recommended number of servings from the food group categories recognized by the DASH and Mediterranean diets. In addition, this section will include healthy recommendations for each of the food group categories as well as calorie values of various foods to assist you in selecting the best food options to maximize your health promoting nutrition and weight loss efforts.

Finally, information to help you become knowledgeable about how to read a food label is provided as part of your behavioral change education.

❑ **Step 6**: Become an expert in the use of the **Daily Nutrition & Activity Record and Weekly Reflection Form**. These records/forms are where you will record the essential information specific to calories consumed in comparison to calories burned. *Because successful weight loss and weight management is based on the principle of effectively managing calories consumed with calories burned, not counting calories of the foods and beverages you consume is like trying to manage your finances without knowing how much money you make and how much money you spend.* As you record these values/amounts your knowledge of what constitutes good and healthy nutrition is enhanced as is your self-awareness of your behavioral patterns of food selections and physical activity.

Forms are provided for 8 weeks of self-monitoring/recording; sufficient time to learn the skills and strategies necessary to empower you to continue your progress forward toward reaching your weight loss and wellness goals. (See page 45)

❑ **Step 7**: This section contains some of the tools of the trade as it comes to successful weight management. Various **Sample Menus** are included to give you an idea as to how to put together a daily menu. (See page 114) Space is also provided for you to create your own menus with the associated calorie values for all items on your menu. **Weekly Shopping Lists** are provided to assist you in purchasing the foods that you will plan to consume for the coming week. (See page 122) In addition, a place to list various health, nutrition, calorie, and weight management resources/websites that you discovered during your process of gaining knowledge is provided. Your developed list becomes a ready reference for continued growth in knowledge and skills to help you better govern your own life in your new and exciting lifestyle of health and wellness. (See page 139)

❑ **Step 8**: Once you have achieved significant behavioral changes, improved your lifestyle, experienced success, and are well on your way to change and becoming – **pass it forward.** Extend yourself to others, share your success, your new knowledge and skills, teach and mentor them along their own path to success. What an enjoyable experience this can be and what a wonderful way to express your gratitude for the goodness and success you have achieved.

# Step 1

# Personal Awareness and Readiness for Change Assessment Tool

In the "Welcome to Your Personal Weight Management and Wellness System" of this book you were asked the question as to whether you had reached a point in your life where you were truly ready to make meaningful lifestyle changes toward achieving your personal weight management and wellness goals. You were informed that most people come to this point in their life after having experienced a "significant life event" or a "moment of intense realization" that stirred their emotions and created in them a deep rooted motivation and initial momentum to press forward in their desires to do whatever was needed to achieve success. Finally, it was emphasized that an individual's personal commitment and diligence to learning and applying true and correct principles would be essential to making the changes necessary for success.

What follows in this Personal Awareness and Readiness for Change Assessment Tool, is a self-administered evaluation designed to 1) increase your relevant awareness as to how your current lifestyle behaviors and attitudes may be affecting your health and quality of life, 2) to assess your motivation and confidence levels in your ability to ***act*** for yourself in making meaningful lifestyle change, and 3) to identify any significant barriers you may currently have to overcome in making meaningful lifestyle change.

Carefully ponder each question, analyze its meaning and application to your life, and then respond as accurately as possible as part of your self-evaluation of readiness for change. This process, done right, can be fun and enlightening and may reveal attitudes and attributes from which to set goals and implement specific strategies.

## Weight Management History

1. Have you attempted to lose weight previously? ❑ Yes ❑ No If yes, what kinds of programs and strategies (interventions that are very precise and measurable) have you done in the past to change your nutritional/eating patterns to lose weight?

    ______________________________

    ______________________________

    ______________________________

2. If you have attempted to lose weight previously, what were the primary challenges/difficulties you experienced in your weight loss efforts? Check all that apply.

    a. _____ A busy schedule that inhibited nutritional preparations, exercise, etc.

    b. _____ Lack of support from spouse, friends, associates, etc.

    c. _____ Lack of nutritional knowledge and weight loss principles

    d. _____ Inability to manage hunger and impulse eating

    e. _____ Lack of prior preparation for potential obstacles

    f. _____ Not really motivated to commit to the requirements of a program

    g. _____ Unwillingness to consistently restrict food/calorie consumption

    h. _____ Unwillingness to consistently engage in exercise

    i. _____ Physical ailments/injuries that impacted your ability to exercise

    j. _____ Other. Please list below:

    ______________________________

    ______________________________

## Lifestyle – Nutrition and Eating Behaviors

1 Do you typically eat breakfast? ❑ Yes ❑ No If yes, what is a typical breakfast for you?

______________________________________________

2. What is a typical snack for you? ______________________________

3. How many refined sugar beverages (8 oz) do you typically consume per day? __________

4. What do you consider your greatest challenge(s) to healthy eating?

______________________________________________

5. Do you consciously strive to drink sufficient amounts of water each day as part of your nutritional efforts? ❑ Yes ❑ No If yes, what do you consider an appropriate amount for you to drink each day?

____ 1-2 cups ____ 3-5 cups ____ 6-8 cups ____ 8+ cups

6. On a scale of 1 to 5 (1=None and 5=Very Knowledgeable), how well do you know the recommended standards for healthy eating and nutrition? Circle your response: 1 2 3 4 5

7. On a scale of 1 to 5 (1=None and 5=Very Knowledgeable), how would you rate your knowledge of proper nutrition as it pertains to weight loss? Circle your response: 1 2 3 4 5

8. On a scale of 1 to 5 (1=None and 5=Very Knowledgeable), how well do you know how to properly prepare foods so they are healthy and low in calories? Circle your response: 1 2 3 4 5

9. On a scale of 1 to 5 (1=Not Willing and 5=Absolutely Willing), how willing are you to make significant changes in your nutritional/eating patterns? Circle your response: 1 2 3 4 5

10. On a scale of 1 to 5 (1=Not at All Ready/Prepared and 5=Absolutely Ready/Prepared), how ready/prepared are you to make changes in your nutritional eating patterns?
Circle your response: 1 2 3 4 5

## Lifestyle – Fitness and Exercise Behaviors

1. Do you currently exercise on a regular basis? ❑ Yes ❑ No If yes, what does your exercise regimen consist of? Check all that apply and circle the specific type if listed.

   a. _____ Cardio – walking, jogging, aerobics, cycling, swimming, rowing, stair stepping, etc.

   b. _____ Resistance training – free weights, machines/equipment, bands, etc.

   c. _____ Sports participation. Preference: ______________________________

2. How many hours per day on average do you spend in *"sitting time"*?

   ____ 0-4 ____ 4-6 ____ 6-8 ____ 8+

   Of these, how many are required for your job or for school work? __________

3. Do you have any physical limitations that would impact your ability to engage in an exercise regimen? ❑ Yes ❑ No If yes, can this limitation be overcome or can an effective alternative activity be substituted? ❑ Yes ❑ No Comment: ______________________________

4. On a scale of 1 to 5 (1=None and 5=Very Knowledgeable), how well do you know the recommended standards (frequency, intensity, and duration) of exercise needed to help prevent disease and improve health? Circle your response: 1 2 3 4 5

5. On a scale of 1 to 5 (1=None and 5=Very Knowledgeable), how well do you know the recommended standards (frequency, intensity, and duration) of exercise for weight loss and weight maintenance efforts? Circle your response: 1 2 3 4 5

6. On a scale of 1 to 5 (1=Not Willing and 5=Absolutely Willing), how willing are you to participate in a regular exercise program? Circle your response: 1 2 3 4 5

7. On a scale of 1 to 5 (1=Not at All Ready/Prepared and 5=Absolutely Ready/Prepared), how ready/prepared are you to incorporate a daily exercise program into your routine? Circle your response: 1 2 3 4 5

## Lifestyle – Other Behaviors

1. On average, how many hours of sleep do you get each night?

   ____ Less than 5 hours ____ 5-6 hours ____ 6-8 hours ____ More than 8 hours

2. How often do you eat out each week? ______________ When you do eat out where do you typically eat? ______________________________

3. Do you have a spouse or friend(s) that would be supportive of your weight management efforts while participating in this program? ❑ Yes ❑ No If no, identify your plans to address this issue. ______________________________

   ______________________________

   ______________________________

4. On a scale of 1 to 5 (1=Poorly and 5=Effectively), how well do you feel you handle stress? Circle your response: 1 2 3 4 5. If you scored yourself anything less than "4" would you say that your response to stress hinders your weight management efforts? ❑ Yes ❑ No If yes, what can you do now to more effectively manage your stress so that it is not a hindrance to your efforts? ______________________________

   ______________________________

   ______________________________

5. On a scale of 1 to 5 (1=Ineffective and 5=Very Effective), how effective do you feel you are at planning ahead, organizing your efforts, and effectively using your time toward reaching your goals? Circle your response: 1 2 3 4 5. If you scored yourself anything less than "4" what adjustments could you make in your life to more effectively maximize your time and efforts toward your weight loss goals?

   ______________________________

   ______________________________

   ______________________________

6. On a scale of 1 to 5 (1=Weak and 5=Strong), how would you rate yourself in your ability to effectively put forth real sacrifice and endure some discomfort (e.g. hunger) as part of working on challenging tasks? Circle your response: 1 2 3 4 5. If you scored yourself anything less than "4" what has kept you from a willingness to give up something or to work to overcome a challenge? ______________________

______________________

What adjustments are you willing to make to satisfy the need for sacrifice in accomplishing your goals?______________________

______________________

7. Express in words your real reason(s) for wanting to lose weight and incorporate a wellness oriented lifestyle at this time in your life. ______________________

______________________

______________________

______________________

## Review and Assessment

Now that you have completed the survey portion of this "tool" you should have an increased awareness of how your current lifestyle, behaviors and attitudes may have impacted your life to this point as it pertains to your health and weight. Hopefully, it also helped you to assess your personal readiness for making significant lifestyle changes, or maybe more importantly, helped motivate and coach you along toward personal readiness.

To that end, and as you look toward your future, are you ready and committed to do what is required to put forth the effort and sacrifice to truly make this your time and season for change?

❑ Yes – Let's get it done. Move on to step 2. Date: ______________

❑ No – If now is not the time to begin your season of change, what do you feel is needed right now to help move you toward that point, and when do you plan to accomplish that?

______________________

______________________

______________________

______________________

______________________

# Step 2
# Establish Your Baseline Health and Fitness Values

Before embarking on your journey of change and becoming, take the time to obtain some basic measurements that will serve as baseline values from which you can measure progress and set goals. Knowing some key physical measurements can provide motivation as you look back upon your progress and experience the realization that your hard work and dedication has paid off in new and improved measurements – the becoming of a new you.

**Initial Assessment Date**: ______________________

## Essential Anthropometric Baseline Measurements

**Height:** ____________ in **Weight:** ____________ lbs

**Body Mass Index** (BMI):
(weight in lbs x 703) ÷ height in inches$^2$

(______ x 703) = _______ ÷ ______ in$^2$

= __________ (BMI)

| BMI | Wt. Status |
|---|---|
| *Below 18.5* | *Underweight* |
| *18.5 – 24.9* | *Normal* |
| *25 – 29.9* | *Overweight* |
| *30 & Above* | *Obese* |



**Waist Circumference:** __________ inches
-Taken at the smallest part of the waist or 2 cm above the umbilicus.

Note: A waist circumference of ≥ 40 inches for males and ≥ 35 inches for females is associated with a high risk for heart disease and Type II diabetes.

**Hip Circumference**: __________ inches
-Taken at the apex of the buttocks and/or directly over the femur bone that can be felt at the lateral side of the hip.

## Other Important Health & Fitness Measurements

These measurements will need to be taken by individuals (wellness coaches, personal trainers, etc.) trained in their assessment protocols and who can provide the appropriate "rating classification" based on the results.

**Percent Body Fat**: ______ %
Rating: ____________________
- Triceps skinfold: ________ mm
- Chest skinfold: ________ mm
- Abdomen skinfold: ________ mm
- Suprailiac skinfold: ________ mm
- Thigh skinfold: ________ mm

**Cardiorespiratory (VO2max)**: ________ ml/kg/min
Rating: ____________________

### Muscular Fitness

**Muscular Endurance**

**Push-ups**: ________ **Ab Curl-ups**: ________
Rating: ____________ Rating: ____________

**Muscular Strength** (1 rep. max)

**Bench Press**: ______ lbs **Leg Press**: ______ lbs
Rating: ____________ Rating: ____________

**Flexibility** (Sit-and-Reach Test): ________ cm
Rating: ____________________

## Selected Cardiovascular Health Measurements

**Blood Cholesterol Values**:

| | | Rec. Value |
|---|---|---|
| • Total Cholesterol: | ________ mg/dL | (<200) |
| • LDL Cholesterol: | ________ mg/dL | (<100) |
| • HDL Cholesterol: | ________ mg/dL | (>60) |
| • Triglycerides: | ________ mg/dL | (<150) |
| • TC/HDL Ratio: | ________ to 1 | (≤3.5 to 1) |

**Resting Heart Rate**:
Beats Per Minute: ________ BPM

**Blood Pressure**:

| | | Recommended Value |
|---|---|---|
| Systolic: | ________ mmHg | (<120) |
| Diastolic: | ________ mmHg | (<80) |

## Your Weight Loss Graph

In this grid, graph your weight loss progress week to week, preferably weighing yourself on the sam day each week and at the same time each day. As you make progress along your path, take time to enjoy seeing your progress in graph form as a nice looking downward trend can serve as a strong motivator to continue your efforts toward your goals.

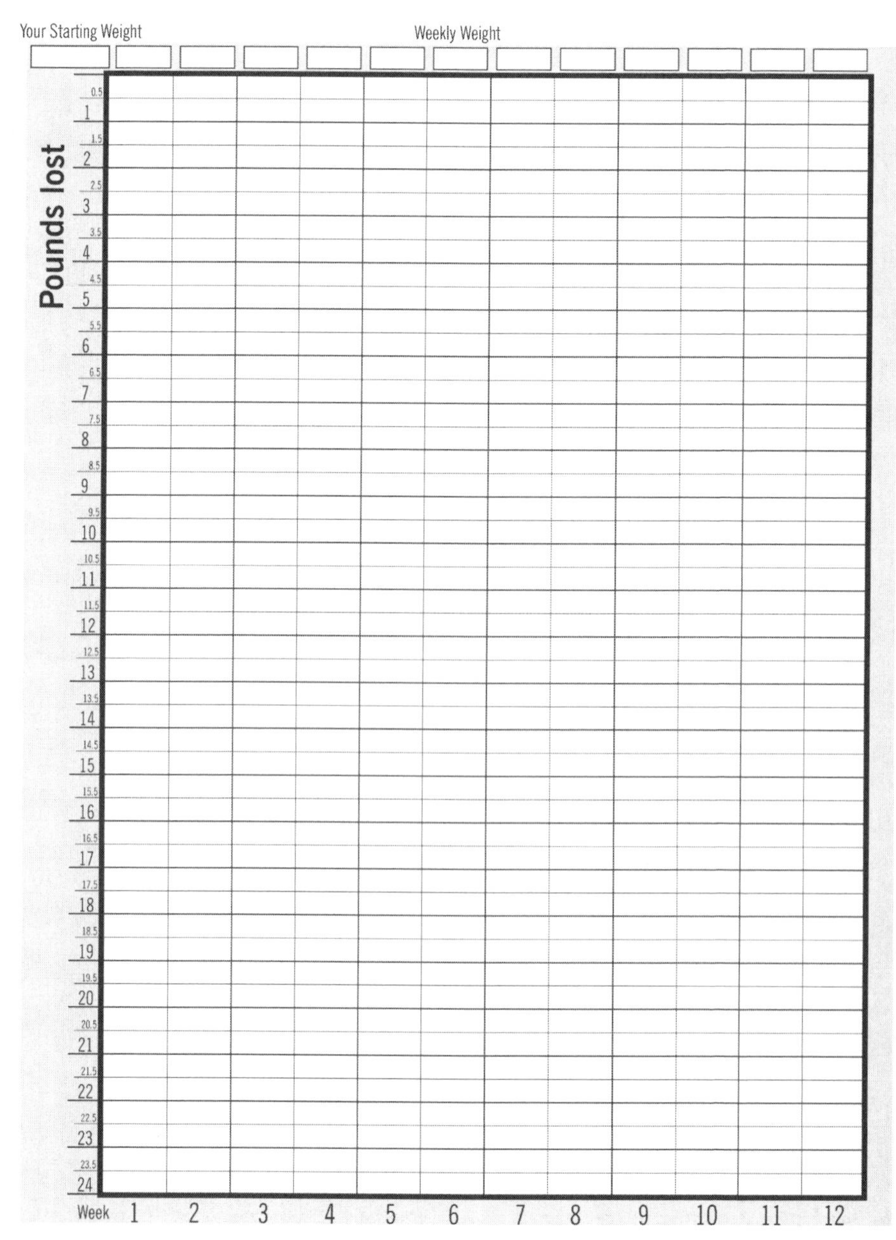

# Step 3

## Setting Goals For Your Journey Ahead

## Recording, Reviewing, Committing, Acting, Becoming, Rewarding

The process of weight loss can be long and fraught with obstacles. Of course, there will be times that are challenging to you and you will experience some discomfort as you change from counterproductive behavioral patterns of the past to the new and exciting health promoting behaviors that are the hallmark of a wellness oriented lifestyle. It will require some sacrifice on your part; be glad for it as it represents your doing something good and worthwhile.

Prepare ahead each day and work a consistent goal oriented plan knowing that you will prevail. Know it in your mind and in your heart, with an understanding that nothing will stand in your way. You have already made the decision, now set the goals – short term and long term – and ***act*** according to true and correct principles to guide the way.

Goals properly established, help keep us focused and motivated. They should be measurable, realistic, and achievable. There is no purpose in setting goals that are so difficult to be achieved that they lead to frustration and discouragement. **Record** your goals as a permanent record of what it is you are working to achieve. **Review** them periodically as an ever present reminder of the purpose of your journey. **Commit** yourself to the line-upon-line efforts required for success and ***act*** in meaningful and productive ways. As you do so you are **becoming** the wellness oriented person who seeks to maximize personal potential through appropriate change. Finally, **reward** yourself for goals successfully achieved as an acknowledgement of your success. Note: There may be times on your journey that you need to re-evaluate or modify your goals as your knowledge and understanding grows of true and correct principles.

### My Body Weight

Target Date

Long Term Goal: ____________________ /________

Short Term Goals:

____________________ /________

____________________ /________

____________________ /________

Reward: ____________________

### My Fitness

Target Date

Long Term Goal: ____________________ /________

Short Term Goals:

____________________ /________

____________________ /________

____________________ /________

Reward: ____________________

### My Nutrition

Target Date

Long Term Goal: ____________________ /________

Short Term Goals:

____________________ /________

____________________ /________

____________________ /________

Reward: ____________________

### My Health, My Life

Target Date

Long Term Goal: ____________________ /________

Short Term Goals:

____________________ /________

____________________ /________

____________________ /________

Reward: ____________________

# Step 4

# Gaining Knowledge and Understanding Essential to Your Success

Included in this section are some key laws and principles, proven strategies and interventions, and demonstrated examples of success that you should understand to successfully manage your weight in an empowered way. Study the material, learn and understand the principles, and then effectively **act** upon them in this your season of change and becoming.

## A Law to be Understood and a Principle for Success

There are certain scientific laws that govern the "how" and "what" of energy use. A proper understanding of the **1st Law of Thermodynamics** is essential knowledge in the effective management of one's body weight. It states that *energy can neither be created nor destroyed; only changed form one form to another.* Simply said, when we gain fat it is because we have consumed more calories (energy) than we have burned. When we lose fat it is because we have burned more calories (energy) than we have consumed. If our weight stays the same it is because the number of calories we have consumed is equal to the number of calories we have burned.

With this understanding it is important to note that one pound of human body fat is equivalent to or provides **3,500 calories**. If, for example, in a given time period (week, month, etc.) we gain one pound of body fat it is because during that time period we consumed 3,500 calories more than we burned. Likewise, if we lose one pound of body fat in a given week it is because we burned 3,500 calories more than we consumed that week. If we lose two pounds of body fat in a given week it is because we burned 7,000 calories more than we consumed that week (7,000/3,500 = 2). This caloric deficit where more calories are burned than consumed in a given time period is known as a **negative energy balance**.

Therefore, if you want to lose weight you must create a negative energy balance. The most effective and appropriate way to accomplish this is to combine a moderate reduction in the calories you eat each day with an increase in the amount of calories you burn through **planned exercise** and basic daily tasks like showering, dressing, household chores, basic office or school work, etc. These basic daily activities are referred to as **Activities of Daily Living** (ADL) and may account for a considerable amount of calories burned each day. Unfortunately, for many people the availability of modern technologies and conveniences have reduced the number of calories burned from their activities of daily living, but this need not be the case. Finally, our bodies also burn a significant number of calories as part of its **Resting Metabolic Rate** (RMR), or the number of calories burned in a 24-hour period while at rest to maintain normal biological functions needed to sustain life. More will be discussed on this later in this book as it plays an integral part of the body's energy equation and in calculating one's customized nutritional plan.

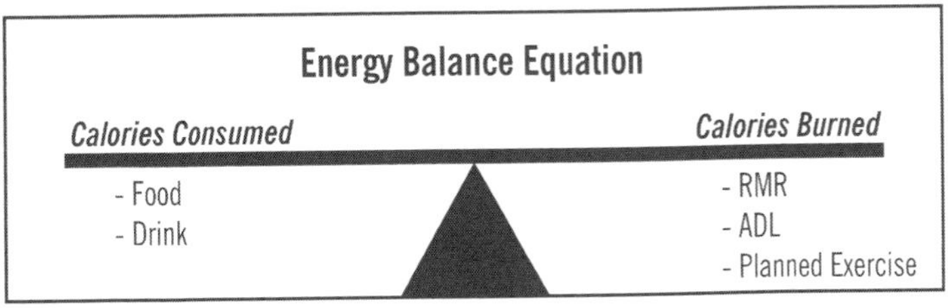

**Energy Balance Equation**

| *Calories Consumed* | *Calories Burned* |
|---|---|
| - Food | - RMR |
| - Drink | - ADL |
| | - Planned Exercise |

The nutritional program of this system is designed to create a moderate reduction in dietary calories, while eating a health promoting balance of nutritious foods from the prescribed food groups. Weight loss achieved without also promoting healthy nutrition makes no sense, can be detrimental to your health and will almost certainly be short lived. As previously mentioned, further adding to the negative energy balance, and thus increasing the weight loss achieved, will come from the calories you burn during planned exercise as well as an increase in calories burned from your activities of daily living. Ultimately, this system, if ***acted*** upon correctly, will help you establish lifelong learning and appropriate behavioral lifestyle changes that promote achieving and maintaining a healthier, leaner, and more efficient body. One that is more capable of going and doing those things that are meaningful to you and which bring you joy and happiness.

Because creating a negative energy balance involves both a reduction in calories consumed and an increase in calories burned, effectively applying the **Principle of Summation** is essential in helping to achieve this negative energy balance. Here is how it works. Let's say that you currently drink 2% milk which contains approximately 5 grams of fat (1 gram of fat = 9 calories) and you consume 2 cups per day. As part of a behavior change strategy you decide to switch to skim milk which is virtually fat free, and yet still drink the 2 cups of milk per day. Because of this change in the type of milk you drink you have effectively reduced the total amount of calories in your milk consumption by 90 calories per day (2 glasses at 5 grams of fat each = 90 calories). Do this for 12 weeks and you have effectively reduced your calorie intake by 7,560 calories (90 calories x 7 days per week x 12 weeks = 7,560) which would result in a loss of 2.16 pounds (7,560 calories/3,500 = 2.16). Not bad for simply making a change in the type of milk consumed without even reducing the amount of milk consumed.

Now let's *add* to (the Principle of Summation) that reduction of calories by increasing the calories burned by simply walking an additional 10 minutes per day. Maybe this could come from a noon walk while eating your lunch or by parking further from work so that it requires you to walk 5 minutes more to and from your car each day. As an example we will consider a 150 pound (68 kg) person walking at a pace of 3.5 miles per hour. In 10 minutes of walking this person would burn approximately 49 calories (the formula for calculating calories burned from activity/exercise is located later in this book). By simply walking an additional 10 minutes 5 days a week this person would burn 245 calories a week due to this simple increase in walking time (49 x 5 = 245). If done for 12 weeks it would total 2,940 calories and yield a weight loss of .84 pounds (2,940/3,500 = .84).

If you *add* these two simple lifestyle changes together they yield a total weight loss in 12 weeks of 3 pounds (2.16 + .84 = 3). Now consider the significance of contribution to your weight loss efforts if you engage in several similarly small activities/strategies aimed at contributing to your efforts to create a greater negative energy balance. There are numerous ways to do this and they all are part of the Principle of Summation. Collectively they can contribute greatly to your overall weight loss goal and wellness oriented lifestyle. Imagine the potential if you add several of these simple strategies to your customized nutritional weight loss plan and regularly scheduled exercise program, all focused on helping you to eat healthy and lose weight effectively. So, be creative and use your own genius to identify several strategies that you can add to your line-upon-line process of change and capitalize on the benefits of the Principle of Summation in your wellness and weight management pursuits.

Another strategy to consider in the Principle of Summation:

Let's say you are an avid pop drinker consuming four 12-ounce cans of pop a day, each containing 140 calories. That's 560 calories consumed each day that provides you no nutritional value, only empty calories that are contributing to your weight gain. Now, as part of your lifestyle behavior change efforts you decide to eliminate two of these cans of pop each day and switch one to a calorie free choice. So, with eliminating two cans of pop each day and replacing one with a calorie free option you have effectively reduced your daily calorie consumption by 420 calories. Multiply this out over a year (assuming everything else remains constant in your life) and you have effectively eliminated 153,300 calories (420 x 365 = 153,300) over the year for a total weight loss of 43.8 pounds (153,300/3,500 = 43.8). Wow! Are you beginning to see the power of the Principle of Summation and how you might make it work for you in your weight management efforts? The possibilities are vast and the benefits exciting.

Now let's consider this principle inversely. Let's say that each day for the next 20 years you only eat 20 calories more each day than you consume (e.g. the amount in a single cracker), but you do it each and every day of those 20 years. At the end of 20 years you will have consumed an additional (beyond what you burned) 146,000 calories for a weight gain of 41.7 pounds (20 x 365 x 20 = 146,000/3,500 = 41.7). This little example demonstrates the importance of calorie counting and is quite interesting when you consider that the average American gains 40 pounds between the ages of 20 and 40.

Can you see how managing your calorie intake and output is essential to your efforts to effectively manage your weight?

## A Demonstration of Success and Lessons to be Learned

There are a number of weight loss programs, systems, fads, etc. that promote the idea that you need not "count calories" to be successful in managing your weight. However, because successful weight loss and weight management is based on the principle of properly managing calories consumed with calories burned, not counting calories is like trying to manage your finances without knowing how much money you make and how much money you spend. **Counting calories** is simply essential baseline knowledge if you are to act in a meaningful and effective way in managing your weight. Equally important is the fact that counting calories requires you to actually learn the caloric value of the foods you eat. This new knowledge allows you to ***act*** in making better food choices and as a result you are exercising wisdom, an attribute that will be essential in navigating your way toward successful and permanent weight loss and weight maintenance.

Lending further validation of this important principle of counting calories is the fact that a number of key studies looking at **calorie intake reporting** showed that subjects under reported the actual number of calories they consumed in a day by an average of 1,000 calories in the study by Skov, by 1,200 calories in the study by Heymsfield, and by 1,453 calories in the study by Buhl.

Skov AR, et al. *Normal levels of energy expenditure in patients with reported "low metabolism."* Clinical Physiology 1997;17:279-285

Heymsfield SB, et al. *The Calorie: myth, measurement, and reality.* American Journal of Clinical Nutrition 1995;62 (supplement):1034s-41s

Buhl KM. *Unexplained disturbance in body weight regulation: diagnostic outcome assessed by double labeled water and body composition analyses in obese patients reporting low energy intakes.* Journal of the American Dietetic Association 1995; 95:1393-1400.

Potential causes of under reporting of calorie intake discussed in these studies included inadequate calorie knowledge, inaccurate portion estimates, memory disturbances (forgetting), and psychosocial motivation. *As such, **the process of recording what and how much you eat and the number of calories thereof (calorie counting) and then comparing that number to the number of calories you burn in a day is an essential principle in a successful weight management program.***

Fortunately, there is a group of individuals who have effectively and convincingly demonstrated the need for this principle, as well as many others, and can teach us some important lessons pertaining to successful weight management. They belong to an exclusive organization known as the **National Weight Control Registry** (http://www.nwcr.ws/), an organization established to track and learn from those who have successfully lost weight (a minimum of 30 pounds) and have kept that weight off for a significant amount of time (a minimum of 1 year). This organization evolved from a landmark study whose purpose was to gather information from these masters of weight management to identify those lifestyle behaviors associated with their successful weight loss and long-term weight loss maintenance. To that end, 74% of individuals in the Registry used food and activity records to "record the foods eaten and the calories in those foods." In other words, "calorie counting" was an essential component to their success, and therein is an example of a correct principle being ***acted*** upon and an important lesson to be learned.

What other lessons can we learn from these masters of successful weight management on our road to success?

- They weighed themselves at least weekly – immediate feedback on their efforts
- They increased their planned exercise and activities of daily living – burning more calories and further increasing the negative energy balance for enhanced weight loss
- They ate more fruits and vegetables – adding volume to their meals helping to control hunger while keeping calorie amounts low
- They reduced dramatically the amount of time spent *sitting, whether that was in front of a television, computer, etc. – usually time that is not progressing us forward in the pursuit of all our goals and aspirations
- They became very effective in using their own creativity and genius in solving weight management problems when they arose – effective management of the sometimes difficult terrain of weight loss
- They worked to develop and nurture supportive relationships while being assertive about their needs in their weight management efforts

It is our privilege to learn from these masters of weight loss and incorporate these and other proven principles and strategies into our overall personal weight management and wellness system.

**A statistical comparison between the average American and members of the NWCR**

| Average American | NWCR Members |
|---|---|
| 44% ate breakfast regularly | 78% ate breakfast daily (a healthy breakfast) |
| 28 hours of TV watching time each week | 61% watch less than 10 hours of TV per week |
| 46.9% meet aerobic exercise guidelines | 90% exercise approximately 1 hour per day |
| Average caloric intake is 2,757 calories per day | 98% modified their food intake |

*As research continues to investigate the relationship between various lifestyle characteristics and disease and death, one particular point of interest, which happens to also have application to weight loss, is that of the relationship between how much time a person spends sitting each day and how soon they will die, or in other words their life expectancy. One particular study conducted by *Katzmarzyk looked at the relationship between sedentary behaviors and mortality in a representative sample of 17,013 individuals between the ages of 18 to 90 who were followed an average of 12 years. After adjustment for potential confounders, there was a progressively higher risk of mortality across higher levels of sitting time from all causes of death and cardiovascular disease (CVD). The researchers concluded that, "These data demonstrate a dose-response association between sitting time and mortality from all causes and CVD, independent of leisure time activity."

*Katzmarzyk, et al. Sitting Time and Mortality from All Causes, Cardiovascular Disease, and Cancer. Medicine & Science in Sports & Exercise 2009; 998-1005

From the standpoint of weight management, sitting time burns very few calories and may lead to premature death. Therefore, specific to the Principle of Summation, increasing the number of calories we burn each day by simply increasing our activities of daily living and avoiding prolonged sitting time, will not only contribute to our weight loss efforts, but may also help us live longer, healthier lives. So, let's act upon this principle and reap the rewards.

## The Essential Role of Exercise in Successful Weight Loss and Weight Loss Maintenance

Scientific evidence is so profoundly clear that the most successful weight loss programs use a combination of dieting and planned exercise to optimize achieving a negative energy balance. In addition, regular exercise is vitally important in maintaining your new body weight following weight loss. It is important to note that 90% of members of the National Weight Control Registry increased their daily *exercise to approximately 60 minutes a day, with aerobic/cardio activities (e.g. brisk walking, jogging, aerobics, circuit training, dance, cycling, Zumba, etc.) being the primary mode of exercise and resistance training providing important additional benefits.

* Moderate exercise is safe for most people, but it is recommended that you talk with your doctor before starting an exercise program, especially if any of the following apply to you.

1. You have a family history of heart disease and are a male over 45 years of age or a woman over 55 years of age, or have heart disease yourself
2. You experience pressure or pain in your chest, neck, shoulders, or arms during physical activity
3. You sometimes feel faint, lightheaded, have dizzy spells, or experience blurred vision or slurred speech
4. You have two or more risk factors for heart disease. These include high blood cholesterol, high blood pressure, diabetes, current smoker, obese, and sedentary.

While an hour of exercise a day is a worthy and recommended goal to aim for, it usually is a habit and capability that develops overtime as you move along the continuum toward a wellness oriented lifestyle. This is certainly understandable and validates the principle that success breeds success. As you experience the benefits of exercise toward your weight loss goals, i.e. enhanced weight loss, you become more motivated to reach a little deeper and push a little harder in your efforts. To maximize the benefits of exercise for weight loss, many individuals turn to Personal Trainers for professional guidance and to help them stay motivated and focused in their efforts.

What follows below is a summary of relevant scientific literature on the role of exercise in one's weight loss efforts. This evidence will no doubt convince you of the essential role of exercise for effective weight loss and weight loss maintenance, but hopefully will also motivate you to incorporate regular exercise into your new wellness oriented lifestyle. The principle of exercise, when regularly practiced enables you with the capacity to go, to do, to become, to serve, to contribute, and to be there for your family and friends with greater vigor.

Studies show that diet + physical activity (PA) weight loss programs resulted in a significantly greater weight loss (-1.1 kg) overall (Shaw et al. 2006). Curioni and Lourenco (2005) reported that diet + PA programs produced a 20% greater weight loss (-13 kg) compared to the diet-only (-9.9 kg) programs as well as a 20% greater sustained weight loss after 1 year. Also, adding exercise to dieting increases the amount of fat lost. Exercise also maintains or slows down the loss of fat free mass (FFM) that occurs with dieting only. Pavlou and colleagues (1985) studied the contribution of exercise to the preservation of FFM in mildly obese males on a rapid weight loss diet. The exercise group dieted and participated in an 8 wk walking-jogging program, 3 days/wk. The nonexercising group dieted only. Although the total weight loss of the exercise (-11.8 kg) and nonexercise (-9.2 kg) groups was similar, the exercise group maintained FFM (-0.6 kg) while the nonexercise group lost a significant amount of FFM (-3.3 kg). For the nonexercising subjects, only 64% of the total weight loss was fat weight compared to 95% for the exercising group.

Similarly, Kraemer and collegues (1999b) compared the effects of a weight loss dietary regiment with and without exercise in overweight men. The diet-only group did not exercise, the exercise groups participated in either an aerobic exercise program or a combined aerobic and resistance training exercise program, 3 days/wk for 12 weeks. By the end of the program all three groups lost a similar amount of weight (-9 to 10 kg), but for the diet only group, only 69% of the total weight loss was fat weight compared to 78% for the diet + aerobic exercise group and 97% for the diet + aerobic + resistance training group.

- **How Exercise Promotes Fat Loss and Preserves Lean Body Mass**
  In response to aerobic and resistance training exercise, levels of growth hormone, epinephrine, and norepinephrine increase. These hormones stimulate the mobilization of fat from storage and activate the enzyme lipase, which breaks down triglycerides into free fatty acids. Free fatty acids are then metabolized and serve as an important energy source, especially during aerobic exercise. Heavy resistance training exercise also stimulates the release of anabolic hormones such as testosterone and growth hormone resulting in increased protein synthesis, muscle growth, and FFM (Kraemer et al. 1991).

- **How Improved Cardiorespiratory Fitness (CRF) Helps Control Body Weight**

  As an individual's CRF level increases through training, the amount of work that the person can accomplish at a given submaximal heart rate increases. Thus, the more fit individual expends calories faster than the less fit individual at a given exercise heart rate. During high-intensity aerobic exercise, lactate production increases and inhibits fatty acid metabolism. However, endurance training increases the lactate threshold (point at which lactate accumulates significantly in the blood). In aerobically trained persons, the percentage of the energy derived from the oxidation of free fatty acids during submaximal exercise is greater than that derived from glucose oxidation (Coyle 1995; Mole, Oscai, and Holloszy 1971). The reduction in muscle glycogen utilization is also associated with a greater rate of oxidation of intramuscular triglyceride (Coyle 1995).

  In order to expend the amount of energy recommended to prevent weight regain after weight loss, cardiorespiratory fitness (VO2max) needs to increase. Therefore, weight reduction programs should increase cardiorespiratory fitness so that participants are able to reach this physical activity goal within a reasonable amount of time (Saris et al. 2003).

- **The Effect of Exercise on Resting Metabolic Rate (RMR)**

  Research indicates that exercise may counter the reduction in RMR that usually occurs as a result of dieting (Thompson, Manore, and Thomas 1996). It is well known that the rate of weight loss declines in the later stages of dieting due to a decrease in RMR. The lowered RMR is an energy-conserving metabolic adaptation to prolonged periods of caloric restriction (Donahue et al. 1984). In a study of 12 overweight females, Donahue and colleagues (1984) reported that diet alone caused a 4.4% reduction in the relative RMR (RMR/BW). After the addition of 8 weeks of aerobic exercise to the program, the relative RMR increased by 5%. The net effect of exercise was to offset the diet-induced metabolic adaptation and return the RMR to the normal, prediet level.

  Exercise may also facilitate weight loss by causing an increase in postexercise RMR. Moderate-to-high-intensity aerobic exercise increases the postexercise RMR by 5% to 16%, and the elevated RMR may persist for 12 to 39 hours postexercise (Bahr et al 1987; Bielinski, Schultz, and Jequier 1985; Sjodin et al. 1996). The postexercise elevation in RMR appears to be related to the exercise intensity and duration (Brehm 1988).

## Estimating Energy (Calorie) Expenditure During Selected Activities

An exercise calorie burn chart with formula for estimating energy (calorie) expenditure during selected physical activities is found below. As you participate in these various activities and use the chart/formula to estimate the number of calories you burn from different exercises, you will gain more knowledge. This knowledge along with the numerous other true and correct principles you wil be learning will magnify your understanding of how to properly manage calories consumed with calories burned.

Note: There are various online exercise calorie burn calculators that can also assist you in knowing how many calories you burn doing given exercises.

As an example, the energy requirement of walking on level ground at a pace of 4.0 mph is equal to 5.0 metabolic equivalents or METS (1 MET = 0.0175 calories x 1 kilogram of body weight x one minute). (***See chart on following page for the MET of selected exercises/activities***). Therefore, if a 180 pound individual (180 pounds/2.2 = 81.8 kilograms) walked at a pace of 4.0 mph he/she would burn 7.1575 calories per minute (0.0175 x 5.0 x 81.8 kg = 7.1575). If this person walked for 30 minutes they would burn a total of 214.7 calories (7.1575 x 30 = 214.7).

**Formula:** 0.0175 **x** METS **x** body weight in kilograms = calories burned per minute of exercise **x** the total number of minutes spent exercising = total calories burned for the exercise.

0.0175 x METS (Activity) x Weight in kg = Calories per min x # Minutes exercising = Total Calories Burned

0.0175 x 8 x 68 kg = 9.52 /min x 60 minutes = 571 Calories burned

0.0175 x METS (Activity) x Weight in kg = Calories per min x # Minutes exercising = Total Calories Burned

0.0175 x ______ x __________ kg = __________ /min x ________ minutes = __________ Calories burned

0.0175 x METS (Activity) x Weight in kg = Calories per min x # Minutes exercising = Total Calories Burned

0.0175 x ______ x __________ kg = __________ /min x ________ minutes = __________ Calories burned

0.0175 x METS (Activity) x Weight in kg = Calories per min x # Minutes exercising = Total Calories Burned

0.0175 x ______ x __________ kg = __________ /min x ________ minutes = __________ Calories burned

0.0175 x METS (Activity) x Weight in kg = Calories per min x # Minutes exercising = Total Calories Burned

0.0175 x ______ x __________ kg = __________ /min x ________ minutes = __________ Calories burned

0.0175 x METS (Activity) x Weight in kg = Calories per min x # Minutes exercising = Total Calories Burned

0.0175 x ______ x __________ kg = __________ /min x ________ minutes = __________ Calories burned

The website below titled, "Compendium of Physical Activities" provides a more comprehensive listing of MET* data for numerous activities and can be accessed to obtain the MET data for exercises/activities not listed in the box on the facing page.

*https://sites.google.com/site/compendiumofphysicalactivities/*

*MET (Metabolic Equivalent): The ratio of the work metabolic rate to the resting metabolic rate. One MET is defined as 1 kcal/kg/hour and is roughly equivalent to the energy cost of sitting quietly. Therefore, the higher the MET of an activity the greater number of calories it will burn in a given time period. A MET also is defined as oxygen uptake in ml/kg/min with one MET equal to the oxygen cost of sitting quietly, equivalent to 3.5 ml/kg/min.

| METS | Activity | Specifications |
|---|---|---|
| 6 | Bicycling | 10-11.9 mph, leisure pace |
| 8 | Bicycling | 12-13.9 mph, moderate pace |
| 10 | Bicycling | 14-15.9 mph, vigorous effort |
| 3 | Bicycling, stationary | 50 watts, very light effort |
| 5.5 | Bicycling, stationary | 100 watts, light effort |
| 7 | Bicycling, stationary | 150 watts, moderate effort |
| 10.5 | Bicycling, stationary | 200 watts, vigorous effort |
| 8 | Conditioning – Circuit Training | Circuit training, including some aerobic movement with minimal rest, general |
| 7 | Conditioning – Rowing | Rowing, stationary ergometer, general |
| 7 | Conditioning – Ski machine | Ski machine, general |
| 4 | Conditioning – Water aerobics | Water aerobics, water calisthenics |
| 9 | Conditioning – Stair stepping ergo. | Stair treadmill ergometer, general |
| 8.5 | Dancing | Aerobic, step, with 6-8 inch step |
| 3 | Home Activities | Cleaning, heavy or major (e.g. wash car, clean garage), vigorous effort |
| 5.5 | Lawn and Garden | Mowing lawn, walk, power mower |
| 7 | Jogging | Jogging, general |
| 8 | Running | Running, 5 mph (12 min/mile) |
| 9 | Running | Running, 5.2 mph (11.5 min/mile) |
| 10 | Running | Running, 6 mph (10 min/mile) |
| 11 | Running | Running, 6.7 mph (9 min/mile) |
| 11.5 | Running | Running, 7 mph (8.5 min/mile) |
| 12.5 | Running | Running, 7.5 mph (8 min/mile) |
| 13.5 | Running | Running, 8 mph (7.5 min/mile) |
| 14 | Running | Running, 8.6 mph (7 min/mile) |
| 15 | Running | Running, 9 mph (6.5 min/mile) |
| 16 | Running | Running, 10 mph (6 min/mile) |
| 8 | Sports – Basketball | Basketball, game |
| 8 | Sports – Intramural football | Football, touch, flag, general |
| 8 | Sports – Frisbee | Frisbee, ultimate |
| 7 | Sports – Racquetball | Racquetball, casual, general |
| 5 | Sports – Baseball or softball | Softball or Baseball, fast or slow pitch, general |
| 3 | Sports –Volleyball | Volleyball, non-competitive, 6 to 9 member team, general |
| 7 | Walking – Backpacking | Backpacking |
| 7 | Walking – climbing hills | Climbing hills with 0 to 9 pound load |
| 6 | Walking – cross country | Hiking, cross country |
| 6.5 | Walking – race | Race walking |
| 2.5 | Walking | Walking, 2.0 mph, level, slow pace, firm surface |
| 3.3 | Walking | Walking, 3.0 mph, level, moderate pace, firm surface |
| 5 | Walking | Walking, 4.0 mph, level, very brisk pace, firm surface |
| 7 | Water Activities | Swimming, backstroke, general |
| 10 | Water Activities | Swimming, breaststroke, general |
| 11 | Water Activities | Swimming, butterfly, general |
| 8 | Water Activities | Swimming, sidestroke, general |
| 8 | Water Activities | Water jogging |
| 8 | Winter Activities | Skiing, cross country, 4.0-4.9 mph, moderate speed and effort |

## Nutrition for Weight Management and Health Protection

Earlier in this book it was stated that "weight loss achieved without also promoting healthy nutrition makes no sense, can be detrimental to your health, and will almost certainly be short lived."

The nutritional component of the Personal Weight Management and Wellness System is derived from evidence-based data obtained from the Dietary Approaches to Stop Hypertension (DASH) Diet and the so called Mediterranean Diet or lifestyle. Both of these programs are based on eating a proper balance of real food, not prepackaged foods and formulations. Reliance on prepackaged foods is an approach that eliminates the essential element of acquiring sound nutritional knowledge and understanding of correct principles that will be needed for you to ***act*** for yourself in making real behavior change toward permanent weight management and lifelong governance of one's self.

The **DASH diet** is an eating plan rich in fruits and vegetables, low to moderate in fat, high in fiber, low-fat or non-fat diary selections, and whole grains – providing a diet rich in potassium, calcium, and magnesium. Originally developed as a healthy nutritional lifestyle for managing high blood pressure, its combination of nutrient dense, yet calorie low foods from a variety of food groups along with an appropriate amount of protein provides an effective intervention for weight loss and health promotion.

The **Mediterranean diet** emphasizes eating primarily plant based foods such as fruits and vegetables whole grains, and legumes and nuts. It replaces butter and margarines with healthy fats such as olive oil and uses herbs and spices instead of salt to flavor foods. It limits red meats while increasing the consumption of fish and poultry. Beverages consumed are high in flavonoids such as red wine and purple grape juice.

Both plans have numerous demonstrated and documented health promotion and disease preventing benefits. "A Time and Season for Change: Personal Weight Management and Wellness System" combines these healthy eating patterns with an evidence-based caloric energy equation to customize (based on your unique resting metabolic rate) your specific nutritional plan calorie level. A caloric deficit (negative energy balance) is calculated to produce a 1-2 pound weight loss each week, "independent of exercise". Then, **every additional calorie you burn during the week as part of your exercise program adds to the overall negative energy balance and yields "additional" weight loss.**

Therefore, the correct and consistent execution of your customized nutritional plan in conjunction with participation in calorie burning exercise is your formula for success – in losing excess body fat and in providing your body with a rich and balanced supply of vitamins, minerals, healthy fats, phytochemicals, and other important nutrients for protection against the major chronic illnesses of our day.

## Behavior Management in Your Season of Change

What follows in this section are a variety of evidence-based principles, recommendations and interventions (strategies, tools, etc.) presented in a concise and abbreviated format that can be of real benefit to you as you seek to modify certain lifestyle behaviors to promote healthy weight loss and to cultivate a culture of wellness in your life. Some of these behavior management interventions, if successfully ***acted*** upon, can have a profound impact toward your success. Others are simpler and less dramatic in their impact, but all can work together for your good. Select a few to experiment on each week. Determine which ones best help you deal with the inherent challenges of weight loss. They can help you address your specific needs, minimize any weaknesses you might have, and magnify your strengths as you navigate your way in this season of change and becoming.

## Social Support – A Source of Strength and Encouragement

It can be very helpful in your journey of change to travel it with someone who will support your efforts and give you encouragement along the way. That person(s) may be your spouse or friend, who may or may not themselves be engaged in their own season of change. It may be someone trained in the knowledge and skills to assist you with your nutrition and fitness and in your problem solving efforts.

The journey is always more enjoyable when you can share it with someone as long as that person is someone you can trust as a source of strength and inspiration to you and your efforts. If your personality and desires are for someone as a social support, determine who that person might be, invite them to join you on the journey (personally or only emotionally) and then go to work and enjoy your season of change together.

## Creating Your Plan and Executing That Plan

Successful people always have a plan to help them accomplish their goals. Their plan consists of several smaller tasks directed toward keeping them on track and overcoming any obstacles that may arise. To be successful at losing weight you need to become an organized, attention to detail, forward thinking, flexible and adaptive kind of person. These characteristics will spill over into all areas of your life and enhance your quality of life and personal accomplishments.

Each day you should **plan ahead for the next day**, especially as it comes to what you will eat and when you will exercise. Build it into your schedule and your mind set. For example, most people eat the same breakfast or a limited variety of breakfast selections each day. Therefore, your breakfast should be "***known***" each day – what and how much you will eat and the total amount of calories for that breakfast. Your lunch and snack(s) should be "***planned***", whether you take your lunch with you so you control what you eat, or what you will purchase at work or school and the amount of calories for that lunch. For this purpose your book provides a few **Sample Menu Plans** (See page 130) specific to your nutritional plan calorie level along with forms on which to develop your own (acting) menu plans or meals specific to your unique food options and preferences. Finally, your end of the day meal will be "***determined***" by how many calories you have remaining toward your nutritional plan calorie level limit for the day. Determine how many calories you still can consume and stay within your calorie limit. Then creatively design a meal that accommodates that limit and helps round out the recommended servings from respective food groups for health promoting nutrition.

At the end of each week you should plan ahead for the next week by shopping for those food items that will facilitate your plan. For this purpose a **Weekly Grocery List** (See page 138) is provided to help you think of those items you need to purchase to be "prepared in all needful things" so that you can execute your plan. Failing to plan ahead leaves you at the mercy of what you happen to have on hand verses what you should have readily available.

Also important is to plan your exercise for the day and any activities of daily living strategies that can help you increase the calories you will burn. For example, know what, when, and how much elevated heart rate exercise you will accomplish for the day and have it built into your routine. Don't let anyone or anything rob you from this important "you time" as it is an investment in you, your health, and your future. Look for ways to increase your activities of daily living a part of how you simply go about your day. For example, if you have the option between an elevator and stairs, choose the stairs and "bounce" up them instead of slowly walking them. Walk a little faster and farther during your lunch or break periods with the understanding that by "sitting" less and walking more you are not only increasing your calorie burn toward weight loss, but may reduce your risk of premature death.

### Positive and Constructive Thinking – The Foundation for *Acting* vs Being Acted Upon

The opposite of positive and constructive thought processes are negative and destructive thinking patterns. Because our thought processes can strongly influence our behaviors it only makes sense that a person who thinks optimistically will approach the process of weight loss with an effective and motivating attitude. An attitude that will work to overcome obstacles, solve problems, see potential, and know that in the end you will be successful. This kind of positive attitude is essential for success.

Negative and flawed thinking, on the other hand, causes us to be acted upon via false and distorted beliefs that only serve to thwart our efforts and lead to frustration and disappointment. Any thought that does not lift, build and edify you and your efforts fits into this category. Why go there when we know that weight loss, while at times is difficult, is more than worth it and has and will be accomplished by thousands. Why not you!

Therefore, our thought processes will be:

- I can do this. I can ***act*** and stop being acted upon. Being acted upon got me here in the first place and now I am ready to ***act*** in meaningful ways to achieve my goals.
- I control my destiny and I am capable of making it a good one.
- This ***acting*** for myself is kind of "cool" and a whole lot better than being acted upon. Man is this worth it!
- I am going to learn from this journey and in the end enjoy a new and changed me, one that is capable of going, doing, and becoming according to my potential.
- Stressful time of life – yeah, but I can effectively manage it and keep my forward progress.
- Any cravings I experience will pass shortly as I execute my new behavioral change knowledge and skills to effectively deal with this or any other challenges that come along.
- I love the self-control and self-governance I am developing in this process and know that I am becoming more and more self-reliant, not only in my weight management efforts, but in every aspect of my life. My success in this is breeding other successes and I love that.
- I could eat that, but I choose not to because I am ***acting*** for myself and I am worth what my diligence will ultimately yield – a new and exciting me.
- I could sit and watch the TV, but I choose to get out and enjoy the privilege it is to use this body of mine as the wonderful gift it was intended to be.
- Wow! I am learning so many new and exciting things about nutrition and fitness and my potential that I can't wait to help others experience this wonderful season of change for themselves.
- When I reach my goals, and I absolutely will, I am going to enjoy my new wardrobe, how I look in the mirror and to others, and my new vigor and vitality to go and do things I have not done in years. Then, I am going to share my success with others and help mentor them along the path – a kind of passing it forward.

## Breakfast – Don't Skip It!

Breakfast is probably the most important meal of the day as it provides your body with the fuel and nutrients to start the day and lays the foundation for day-long and life-long health. "Start right to end right" is a motto that certainly applies to breakfast. Skipping breakfast is associated with a depressed metabolism, increased food consumption throughout the day, and is strongly linked to the development of obesity.

Another important consideration of a good breakfast (and possibly all meals) is the mounting evidence that the combination of a high carbohydrate and protein breakfast may overcome the diet-induced compensatory increases in hunger, craving, and ghrelin levels. Ghrelin is a hormone originating in the stomach, which in elevated levels causes hunger and drives appetite and appeal for high calorie foods. Some evidence even suggests that elevated ghrelin levels may even suppress a body's metabolism.

In a study by D. Jakubowicz et al., 193 obese, sedentary non-diabetic adult men and women (47+ 7 years) were randomized to a low carbohydrate breakfast (LCb) or to a high carbohydrate and protein breakfast (HCPb). After 16 weeks on the program both groups exhibited similar weight loss; 15.1 + 1.9 kg in the LCb group vs 13.5 + 2.3 kg in the HCPb group. However, fasting measured ghrelin levels were reduced after breakfast by 45.2% in the HCPb and only 29.5% in the LCb. Consequently, from week 16 to 32, the LCb group regained 11.6 + 2.6 kg, while the HCPb group lost and additional 6.9 + 1.7kg. Also, satiety was significantly improved and hunger and craving scores were significantly reduced in the HCPb group vs the LCb group.

Therefore, an important strategy in helping to control hunger throughout the day when restricting calories begins with a healthy high carbohydrate and protein breakfast. It may help prevent weight regain by reducing the diet-induced compensatory changes in hunger, craving, and elevated ghrelin.

## Problem Solving – The Fun of Acting

As with periodic setbacks you will also be confronted with sudden surprises – events and circumstances that may cause you to deviate from your planned schedule or routine. For example, say you brought your lunch to work or school and know the number of calories and food group servings of what you prepared. Then, a friend or colleague invites you to lunch and they pick the establishment where you will eat. Suddenly you are faced with a potential problem, or could we say opportunity to use your skills and creativity to adjust your plan. Not only can this be fun, but consider the sense of accomplishment as you strategically and successfully navigate around this potential problem. In so doing you will learn and gain valuable experience as a result of your problem solving efforts.

Or, consider the unexpected alteration to your schedule of planned exercise. Rather than getting frustrated, evaluate your options to adjust your schedule and realize that you may need to divide the planned minutes of exercise up into increments for that day, or over the coming day or two. In other words, not a problem and you have been given the opportunity to ***act*** by having to do some things different than planned. Is not this a big part of life – making adjustments as curves are routinely thrown at us? Embrace these events in your life, put on your sleuth hat, and have fun solving the problems that undoubtedly will arise.

## Winning the Hunger Game – Proven Strategies For Success

Experiencing some hunger on your journey is to be expected. It is also important to understand that this is not hunger that is driven from inadequate nutrition intake for health, but rather from the necessary reduction in calories needed to create a negative energy balance for weight loss. Listed below are a few strategies that have proven helpful in managing the hunger feelings that you might experience.

- **Eat a healthy breakfast**. Leaner people almost always eat breakfast. Breakfast at the end of an all-night fast helps jump start your metabolism for the day that will otherwise remain a bit suppressed. It also helps prevent against the sharply increased hunger and associated excess eating that may result from low blood sugar from having not eaten breakfast.
- Carry a **water bottle** with you virtually all the time and drink from it frequently, especially if you are feeling hungry. Not only can it help curb hunger for a period of time, but provides your body with an essential nutrient for good health.
- Craving sweets? A delicious **fruit, low calorie snack, or a zero calorie drink** can take the edge off of that sense of feeling hungry. Remember, will you be prepared by having these on you because you planned ahead. No unpreparedness.
- Try chewing some **gum** for both flavor and a sense of eating derived from the chewing mechanism.
- Try eating multiple **smaller meals** throughout the day instead of three larger meals a day.
- In your meals and snacks, include **high fiber foods** that create a sense of satiety.
- When experiencing hunger that needs to be addressed (cravings) try a **low calorie healthy food** such as a low-calorie yogurt, celery, or anything that works for you to help curb the craving.
- Drink a glass of water just before eating. Your feeling of hunger might be more that you are thirsty than hungry. Either way, a drink of water can help manage hunger.

## The Inevitable Set Backs – May They Be For Your Good

While on your journey of change, and specific to your weight loss efforts, you will undoubtedly encounter some setbacks. This is simply the nature of the beast. Those setbacks may come in the form of getting distracted and deviating from your nutritional plan, an unexpected change in your daily routine or circumstances that affect the consistency of your routine, a transient return to a dysfunctional thinking pattern that works to diminish your motivation or optimism for success, or an injury that temporarily limits activity. Whatever the reason it doesn't matter. What matters is how you respond to these challenges. If at this time you choose to ***act***, by evaluating the reason for the setback, reminding yourself of the goals you have set and why you want to achieve them, and recommitting yourself to your plan then you can move forward with the same confidence. In fact, many times the things learned as a result of your dealing with the setback can become instrumental in your ability to make appropriate adjustments and ultimately make permanent behavior changes toward success. So, when setbacks come, and they will, learn from them, grow in important ways, and know that the experience can ultimately be for your good. This is your new mind-set. Others have overcome these obstacles and so will you.

### Healthy Eating – What's In Your Budget

When eating on a budget there are many ways to get all you need of good and nutritious foods. Consider the following:

1. Plan your meals and snacks (and needed ingredients) before you go shopping. Make a list using the Weekly Grocery List at the back of this booklet and stick to it avoiding the treacherous impulse buying.
2. Never shop when you are hungry. Therefore, eat a healthy snack and drink a large glass of water beforehand.
3. Go shopping after having completed your exercise routine, when you are keenly aware of the hard work you are performing and the desire to not diminish your efforts.
4. Once a month do a "big shop" day to load up on the essential non-perishable products.
5. Set aside a budget for perishable food such as milk, bread, fruits and vegetables, etc.
6. Pay attention to weekly shopping ads. Plan meals around healthy foods that are on sale that week.
7. Couponing can help you purchase foods at a reduced price. Only purchase foods that you need and will eat.
8. Buying fruits and vegetables – 1) eat what is in season, 2) purchase what is on sale and in bulk if applicable, 3) only buy what is on your list, a little bit at a time so the food does not spoil 4) buy canned or frozen, 5) buy store brand, 6) plant your own garden, and 7) plan and cook "smart".

Planning ahead and making the best selections can indeed allow you to eat healthy on a budget, further empowering you in your doing and becoming.

### Adequate Sleep – An Essential Component of Successful Weight Loss

Some important studies looking at the impact of insufficient sleep on weight loss have shown a reduction in total weight lost, increased hunger, reduced energy expended during activities of daily living (simply moving slower due to being tired), and increases in the levels of Ghrelin in the blood. Ghrelin is a hormone that in higher levels has shown to suppress metabolism, stimulate hunger, and increase glucose production in the body.

As such, if you suffer from inadequate sleep on a consistent basis it is vitally important that you take steps to improve your sleep time. Studies show that regular exercise is an important strategy toward better sleep as it significantly increases restorative REM sleep. This will give you the energy to engage in your daily activities as well as exercise; burning more fat and contributing to a healthier you. Put this to the test and you will experience the benefits of a good night's rest. It will be an investment in yourself where the benefits will be seen and felt.

### Dining Out – 10 Tips to Keep on Track

Dining out need not be a time of set-back in your weight management efforts. Rather, it can be an enjoyable experience to take control of the situation by ***acting*** on knowledge and implementing strategies that keep you on target. Your opportunity is to try one of more of the following and gain the confidence of knowing you are making choices that will be for your good.

1. Plan ahead and select a restaurant that has healthy menu selections that you enjoy.
2. Have in mind a healthy selection before you even open the menu and seek it out.
3. If you are not familiar with a particular menu, thoroughly review all options and chose a meal that helps you meet your food group requirements.
4. Ask the waiter to recommend low fat selections.
5. Be proactive and make special requests such as:
    - Dressings, sauces, creams, etc. on the side or omitted completely
    - An omelet made with only one yolk (or no yolk)
    - Cottage cheese, plain yogurt, or low-calorie salad dressing on baked potatoes
    - Broiled entrees without butter or oil
    - Steamed vegetables
    - Non breaded foods
6. Share an entrée with a friend and save some money as a side benefit.
7. Select water as your drink.
8. Consider choosing an appetizer as your main course.
9. Always look for smaller portion options.
10. At fast food restaurants select smaller burgers, grilled chicken sandwiches or salads with low-calorie dressings, cups of fresh fruit, low-fat milk, or bottled water.

## My Own Behavior Modification Strategies – Those Created By Me, That Work For Me

In this box write those behavior modification strategies that you create and work for you, or that you learn as you continue your learning in this your season of change and becoming.

| | |
|---|---|
| | |
| | |
| | |
| | |
| | |

# Step 5

## Determining Your Nutritional Plan Calorie Level and Food Group Servings

**Step 5a**: Calculate your **Resting Metabolic Rate** (RMR), which is the number of calories your body burns in a 24-hour period while at rest and in the fasting state. It represents the number of calories burned to maintain normal biological functions, e.g. heart contractions, breathing, brain functions, liver, kidney, and other organ processes, muscle tonus, etc. Your RMR serves as the foundational framework from which to construct your nutritional plan to achieve a negative energy balance for effective weight loss. To calculate your RMR you need to know your weight in kilograms (kg), height in centimeters (cm), and your age. The formulas are below.

Your weight in pounds 150 ÷ 2.2 = 68 (weight in kg)

Your height in inches 66 x 2.54 = 168 (height in cm)

### Calculating Your Resting Metabolic Rate (RMR)

**Men:** (10 x weight in kg) + (6.25 x height in cm) – (5 x age) + 5 = RMR

(10 x 68 kg) + (6.25 x 168 cm) – (5 x 21) + 5 = ______ RMR

**Women:** (10 x weight in kg) + (6.25 x height in cm) – (5 x age) - 161 = RMR

(10 x 68 kg) + (6.25 x 168 cm) – (5 x 21) - 161 = 1464 RMR

**Step 5b**: Calculate your **Activities of Daily Living** (ADL) by multiplying your RMR by a factor of 1.25 (the non-exercise activity thermogenesis or NEAT). Your ADL is an estimate of the number of calories you burn performing daily tasks like showering, dressing, household chores, basic office and school work, etc. It does not include calories you burn while doing planned exercise such as fitness walking, jogging, cycling, swimming, resistance training, and playing sports. It also does not include the calories that you might burn at work that is beyond basic office work, e.g. heavy labor, etc. which burns considerable more calories.

### Calculating Your Activities of Daily Living (ADL)

RMR x 1.25 = ADL

1464 x 1.25 = 1830 ADL

**Step 5c**: Calculate Your **Nutritional Plan Calorie Level** (NPCL) by subtracting a determined amount of calories (*between 500 to 1000) from your ADL value. This adjusted calorie intake value represents your customized nutritional plan calorie level that will produce a negative energy balance and cause your body to burn its fat stores to make up the energy difference and thus lead to fat loss.

### Calculating Your Nutritional Plan Calorie Level (NPCL)

ADL – (500 to 1000 calories) = NPCL

1830 - 500 calories = 1330 Nutritional Plan Calorie Level (NPCL)

*A daily negative energy balance of 500 calories will produce a 1 pound weight loss per week; a daily 1000 calorie negative energy balance will yield a 2 pound weight loss per week.

**NOTE**: Going below a daily nutritional plan of 1200 calories is associated with inadequate nutrition and greater loss of lean body mass and should therefore be avoided.

**Step 5d**: Using your Nutritional Plan Calorie Level (NPCL), reference the "**Food Group Servings by Calorie Levels**" chart below for the number of servings you should consume in each food group category based on your specific calorie level. Also note the recommended daily water/fluid intake fo the respective genders.

| Food Group Servings by Calorie Levels | | | | | | | | |
|---|---|---|---|---|---|---|---|---|
| | Calorie Levels→ | | | ↓Daily Servings | | | | |
| ↓Food Group | 1,200 | 1,400 | 1,600 | 1,800 | 2,000 | 2,200 | 2,400 | *Ave. Single Serv. Size Calorie Value |
| Grains | 3 | 5 | 6 | 7 | 8 | 9 | 10 | 80 Calories |
| Fruits | 2 | 2 | 2 | 3 | 3 | 3 | 3 | 60 Calories |
| Vegetables | 3 | 3 | 4 | 4 | 5 | 5 | 6 | 50 Calories |
| Dairy | 3 | 3 | 3 | 3 | 3 | 3 | 3 | 100 Calories |
| Protein | 4 | 4 | 5 | 5 | 5 | 5 | 6 | 55 Calories |
| Legumes | 0.5 | 0.5 | 0.5 | 0.5 | 1 | 1 | 1 | 100 Calories |
| Nuts & Seeds | 0.5 | 1 | 1 | 1 | 1 | 2 | 2 | 90 Calories |
| Fats/Oils | 2 | 2 | 2 | 3 | 3 | 3 | 3 | 45 Calories |
| Water | Men should aim for 12 cups of fluid per day, women should aim for 8 cups per day, with 60% -75% coming from water | | | | | | | |

**Because the calorie amount of various food group single serving options can vary significantly, this calorie level represents the average number of calories for a single serving from that food group. Therefore, try to select food options that when averaged together for the day are near the single serving size calorie value. This will help to ensure that your daily calorie intake does not exceed your NPCL.*

**Step 5e**: Learn what constitutes a single serving for each food group category from the chart below. General examples are listed for what is equivalent to a single serving in the respective food groups.

**1 Serving =**

| Grains | Fruits & Vegetables | Dairy |
|---|---|---|
| -1 slice bread (1 ounce)<br>-1/2 small bagel, bun, muffin (1 ounce)<br>-1 small tortilla, pancake<br>-1/2 to 1 cup dry cereal (1 ounce)<br>-1/2 cup cooked cereal, rice, pasta<br>-3 cups popcorn (air popped)<br>-Crackers (1 ounce) | -1 medium size fruit<br>-1/2 cup fresh, frozen or canned fruit<br>-3/4 cup fruit or vegetable juice (100% Juice)<br>-1 cup raw vegetables<br>-2 cups raw leafy greens (lettuce or spinach)<br>-1/2 cup cooked vegetables<br>-1/2 potato (4 ounces) | -1 cup milk or yogurt (skim or 1%)<br>-1/2 cup cottage cheese<br>-1 1/2 ounces non-fat or part-skim cheese |
| **Protein** | **Legumes** | **Nuts & Seeds** |
| -1 ounce poultry, fish, shell fish, or meat<br>-1 egg (2 egg whites)<br>-1 Tbl. peanut butter | -1/2 cup cooked dry beans/peas or tofu | -1 Tbl. sunflower seeds (1/2 ounce)<br>-2 Tbl. nuts (1/2 ounce) |
| | **Fats/Oils & Condiments** | |
| -1 tsp. oil or soft margarine<br>-1 tsp. regular mayonnaise<br>-1 Tbl. cream cheese<br>-1 Tbl. diet margarine | -1 Tbl. low-fat mayonnaise<br>-1 Tbl. regular salad dressing<br>-2 Tbl. light salad dressing<br>-2 Tbl. regular or light sour cream | -2 Tbl. parmesan cheese<br>-1 Tbl. honey<br>-1 Tbl. jam/jelly |

**Step 5f**: Review the information for each food group category, gaining knowledge of the available selections, their calorie values, and helpful recommendations to maximize their nutritional impact. Then apply this knowledge in the selection of foods that best help you achieve your weight loss and nutritional goals, thus ***acting*** in wisdom.

# Grains

Any food made from wheat, rice, oats, cornmeal, barley or another cereal grain is a grain product. Grains are a major source of dietary fiber, are rich in B vitamins, and provide important minerals and phytochemicals.

**Key Recommendation:** Eat mostly 100% whole grain products.

## Recommendations:

- Look for ways to substitute a whole grain product for a refined one in recipes and menus. For example, try brown rice and whole-wheat pasta
- Use whole grains in mixed dishes such as barley in vegetable soup
- Experiment with substituting whole wheat or oat flour for up to half of the flour in a pancake, waffle, muffin, or other flour-based recipes
- Use whole grain bread or cracker crumbs in meatloaf
- Try rolled oats or crushed, unsweetened whole grain cereal as breading for baked chicken, fish, veal cutlets, etc.
- Use unsweetened, whole grain ready-to-eat cereal as croutons in salad or in place of crackers with soup
- Snack on popcorn
- Choose a whole grain cereal or oatmeal for breakfast in the morning

## What to Look For on the Label:

- Choose foods that name one of the following whole grain ingredients first on the label's ingredient list: brown rice, bulgar, graham flour, oatmeal, whole grain corn, whole oats, whole rye, whole wheat, wild rice
- Use the Nutrition Facts label and choose products with a higher %Daily Value for fiber
- Note: Food labeled with the words "multi-grain", "stone-ground", "100% wheat", "cracked wheat", "seven grain", or "bran" are usually not whole grain products
- Note: Color is not necessarily an indication of a whole grain. Bread can be brown because of molasses or other ingredients

**Grains**

| Calories per Ounce | Grains | Fiber Grams |
|---|---|---|
| 65 | Tortilla-Corn | 2 |
| 70 | Whole Wheat Bread | 2 |
| 78 | Bagels | 1 |
| 78 | White Bread | 1 |
| 78 | Sourdough | 1 |
| 90 | Corn Bread | |
| 92 | Tortilla-flour | 2 |
| 98 | Soft Pretzel | 1 |
| 100 | Croissant | 0.5 |
| 100 | Muffins | 1 |
| 100 | Oatmeal | 2 |
| 100 | Pasta | 1 |
| 101 | Buckwheat | 2 |
| 105 | Rice | 1 |
| 105 | Cereal (boxed) | 1 |
| 107 | Couscous | 1 |
| 110 | Rolls | 0.5 |
| 135 | Barley | 4 |
| 136 | Crackers | 1 |

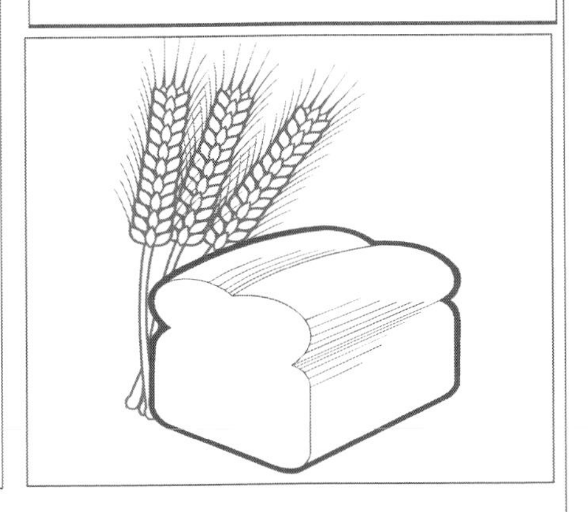

# Fruits

Fruits are rich in compounds known as phytochemicals that provide antioxidants and other health promoting properties against the leading chronic diseases. Because of their sugar content their sweetness provides a satisfying alternative to hunger craving.

**Key Recommendation**: Most fruit servings should come from eating the fruit verses drinking fruit juice.

## Fruit Recommendations:

- Keep a bowl of fruit on the table, counter, or in the refrigerator
- Buy fresh fruit in season when they are less expensive, more flavorful, and nutritious
- Frozen fruit is usually high in nutrition having been frozen shortly after being harvested
- Plan for and top your breakfast cereal with a variety of fruit each morning
- Add fruit to coleslaw or tossed salad
- Try meat dishes that incorporate fruit, such as chicken with apricots or mango chutney
- Make a delicious fruit smoothie by blending fresh or frozen fruit with fat-free or low-fat milk or yogurt
- Substitute applesauce for oil when baking cookies and other baked goods
- Make fresh fruit salads by mixing a variety of fruits and topping with lemon juice to prevent them from turning brown with oxidation
- Incorporate fruit into your "desserts"
- Always take a fruit with you to work or school each day and eat it at a scheduled break time
- If you buy a beverage select 100% fruit juices over soda and sugary drinks

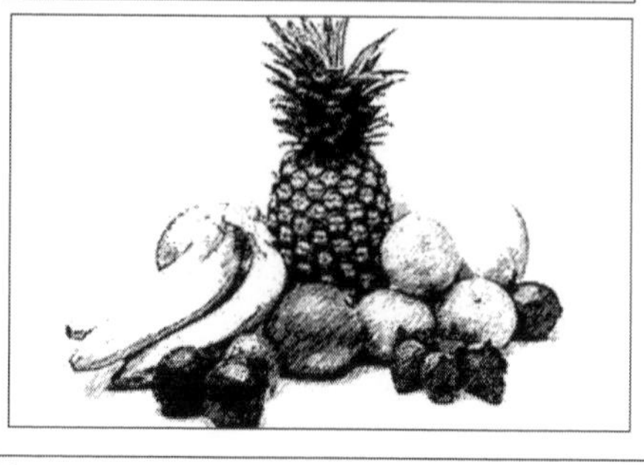

| Fruits | | |
|---|---|---|
| Calories per ½ Cup | Fruit | Fiber Grams |
| 20 | Lime | 2 |
| 23 | Watermelon | 0.5 |
| 25 | Strawberries | 1.5 |
| 26 | Cranberries | 2.5 |
| 27 | Cantaloupe | 1.5 |
| 28 | Papaya | 1 |
| 30 | Honeydew | 1.5 |
| 30 | Nectarines | 1.5 |
| 31 | Blackberries | 4 |
| 31 | Lemon | 3 |
| 31 | Grapes | 0.5 |
| 32 | Raspberries | 4 |
| 33 | Apple | 1.5 |
| 33 | Peaches | 1.5 |
| 37 | Apricots | 1.5 |
| 38 | Plums | 1 |
| 39 | Pineapple | 1 |
| 42 | Blueberries | 2 |
| 43 | Orange | 2 |
| 46 | Cherries | 1.5 |
| 47 | Pear | 2.5 |
| 49 | Grapefruit | 2 |
| 52 | Tangerines | 2 |
| 54 | Mango | 1.5 |
| 55 | Kiwi | 2.5 |
| 67 | Banana | 2 |
| 77 | Olives | 2.5 |
| 120 | Avocado | 5 |
| 157 | Dried Apricots | 5 |
| 197 | Dried Cranberries | 4.5 |
| 204 | Dried Prunes | 6 |
| 217 | Raisins | 3 |
| 250 | Dates | 7 |

# Vegetables

Vegetables are also rich in phytochemicals as well as a variety of vitamins and minerals. They also perform a vital role in efforts to lose excess body fat by providing low calorie options that satisfy hunger, partly because of the healthy amount of protein many contain and partly because of their fiber.

**Key Recommendation**: Most vegetable servings should be the non-starchy type.

## Vegetable Recommendations:

- Wash vegetables prior to preparing/eating them
- Eat a variety of vegetables and experiment by eating those vegetables you have never tried
- Try to incorporate vegetables from the 5 subgroups during the week
- Keep frozen vegetables on hand for quick and easy cooking
- Plan some meals around a vegetable main dish such as stir-fry or soup
- Shred carrots or zucchini into meatloaf, casseroles, quick breads, and muffins
- Include chopped vegetables into pasta sauce or lasagna
- Grill vegetables with meat kabobs
- Add other vegetables to salads
- Add lettuce, tomato, onion, and cucumber to sandwiches, burgers
- Try and eat at least one vegetable for lunch and dinner
- Add vegetables to your egg or omelet
- Keep a bowl of cut up veggies in the refrigerator for snacks

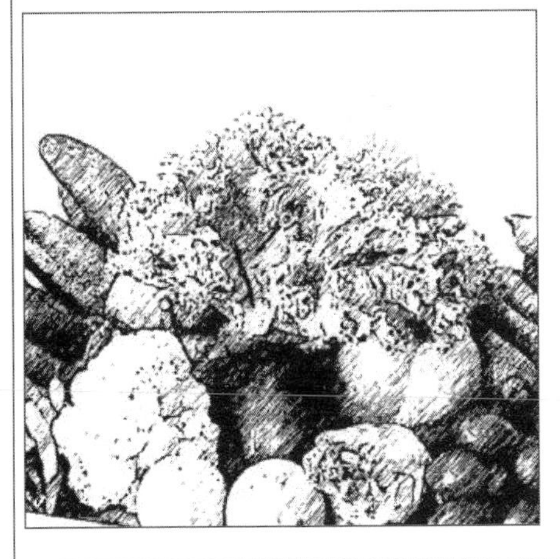

**Vegetables**

| Calories per Cup (raw) | Vegetables | Fiber Grams |
|---|---|---|
| 7 | Spinach | 1 |
| 10 | Lettuce | |
| 11 | Collards | 1 |
| 15 | Mushrooms | 1 |
| 15 | Greens | |
| 16 | Cucumber | 1 |
| 18 | Celery | 1.8 |
| 18 | Turnips | 2 |
| 19 | Green Onions | 1 |
| 19 | Radishes | 1 |
| 20 | Eggplant | 3 |
| 21 | Zucchini | 1 |
| 22 | Cabbage | 2 |
| 24 | Yellow Squash | 1 |
| 25 | Cauliflower | 2.5 |
| 26 | Rhubarb | 2 |
| 27 | Sauerkraut | 4 |
| 27 | Asparagus | 3 |
| 30 | Pumpkin | 3.5 |
| 31 | Broccoli | 2 |
| 34 | Green Beans | 4 |
| 34 | Kale | 1 |
| 35 | Water Chestnuts | 2 |
| 38 | Brussels Sprouts | 3 |
| 38 | Tomatoes | 2 |
| 46 | Jicama | 6 |
| 50 | Rutabaga | 3.5 |
| 52 | Carrots | 4 |
| 54 | Leeks | 1.5 |
| 58 | Beets | 4 |
| 64 | Onions | 3 |
| 86 | Corn | 4 |
| 100 | Parsnips | 6.5 |
| 116 | Potatoes | 3 |
| 117 | Peas | 7 |
| 177 | Yams | 5 |
| 240 | Sweet Potatoes | 4 |

# Dairy

Calcium rich dairy products help protect against osteoporosis by helping build and maintain strong bones. People who consume at least 3 servings of dairy foods each day tend to have lower body mass indexes (BMI).

**Key Recommendation**: Choose dairy products that are non-fat or low-fat.

## Recommendations:

- If you usually drink whole or 2% milk, gradually switch to fat-free milk to lower saturated fat and calorie intake
- Have a fat-free or low-fat yogurt as a snack
- Make a dip for fruits and vegetables from yogurt
- Make fruit smoothies using fat-free or low-fat yogurt
- Craving cheese? Eat a light string cheese as a snack
- Top a baked potato with fat-free or low-fat yogurt or cottage cheese
- Pour fat-free milk over your cold cereal instead of a higher fat content milk
- If you are lactose intolerant, choose lactose-free alternative cheese, yogurt, milk, or soymilk

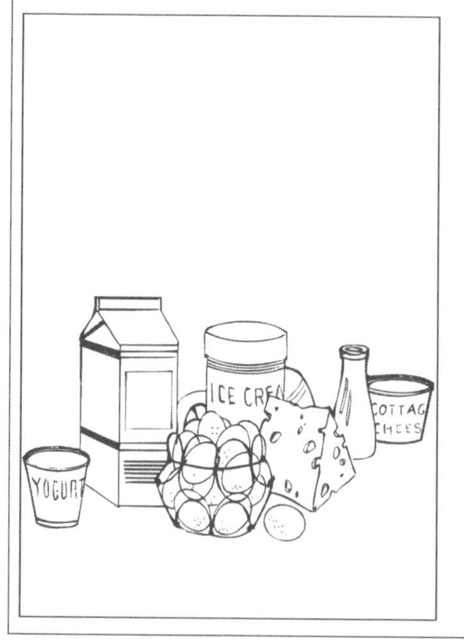


### Dairy

| Calories per Ounce | Cheese |
|---|---|
| 28 | Cottage Cheese |
| 30 | Cream Cheese (non fat) |
| 39 | Ricotta |
| 65 | Cream Cheese (low fat) |
| 72 | Mozzarella |
| 75 | Feta |
| 97 | Cream Cheese (regular) |
| 100 | Provolone |
| 101 | Edam |
| 106 | Havarti |
| 106 | Monterey Jack |
| 108 | Swiss |
| 111 | Parmesan |
| 112 | Colby |
| 114 | Cheddar |

| Calories per Cup | Milk |
|---|---|
| 80-90 | Skim Milk |
| 102 | 1% Milk |
| 122 | 2% Milk |
| 149 | Whole Milk |
| 160 | Yogurt (plain) |
| 80-200 | Yogurt (soft-serve) |
| 160-220 | Cottage Cheese |
| 180-400 | Yogurt (frozen) |
| 192-344 | Eggnog |
| 220-680 | Ice Cream |
| 320 | Half-n-Half |
| 480 | Light Cream |
| 824 | Heavy Cream |

# Protein

Dietary protein provides the building blocks (amino acids) for muscles, bones, blood, skin, hair, nails, organs, hormones, antibodies, and more. Protein provides a lean body mass sparing effect during weight loss as well as helps in hunger management.

**Key Recommendation**: Consistently consume both low-fat or medium-fat protein options, and limit consumption of red meat.

## Selection Tips:

- Boneless chicken breasts and turkey cutlets are the leanest poultry choices
- Fish – select fish rich in Omega-3 fatty acids, such as salmon, trout, mackerel, cod, and herring
- Choose lean or low-fat meats
  Beef: round steaks, roasts (round eye, top round, bottom round, round tip), top sirloin, and chuck shoulder
  Pork: pork loin, tenderloin, center loin, and ham
  Ground beef: extra lean
- Minimize saturated fat and cholesterol in protein selections by choosing egg whites, limiting liver and organ meats
- Experiment with a veggie burger and liven it up with spices and vegetables
- If you are a bacon lover, try turkey bacon

## Preparation Tips:

- Remove skin from poultry before cooking/eating
- Trim all visible fat from meats before cooking
- Broil, grill, roast, poach, or boil meat, poultry, or fish instead of frying
- Choose and prepare foods without high fat meat based sauces or gravies

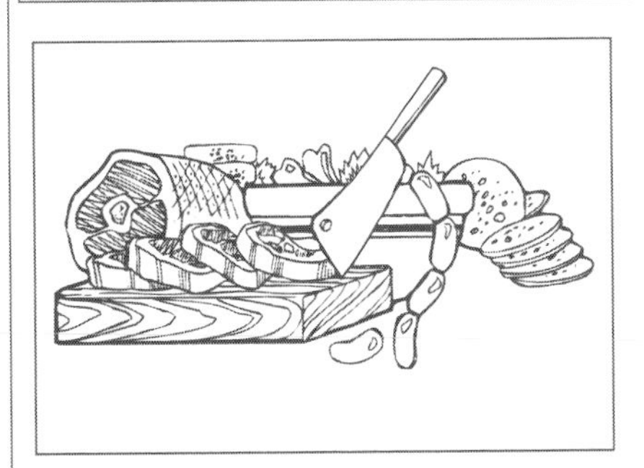

| Protein | |
|---|---|
| Calories per Ounce "cooked" | Fish, Poultry, Shell Fish, Meat |
| 25 | Lobster |
| 27 | Crab |
| 28 | Snapper |
| 30 | Cod |
| 31 | Halibut (Atlantic/Pacific) |
| 33 | Tuna (water packed) |
| 34 | Shrimp |
| 40 | Poultry (light, skinless) |
| 42 | Clams |
| 42 | Trout |
| 45 | Oysters |
| 46 | Veal |
| 49 | Mussels |
| 53 | Tuna (oil packed) |
| 53 | Halibut (Greenland) |
| 54 | Turkey |
| 58 | Sirloin Steak |
| 60 | Pork Spare Ribs |
| 60 | Salmon |
| 65 | Catfish |
| 65 | Poultry (dark, skinless) |
| 66 | Pork Chop |
| 72 | Egg (whole raw) |
| 82 | Ham |
| 84 | Ground Beef |
| 88 | T-Bone Steak |
| 93 | Beef Sausage |
| 95 | Pork Sausage |
| 115 | Prime Rib |
| 130 | Bacon |

# Legumes

Legumes are considered part of the protein food group, but are listed here separately to draw attention to their important health benefits and need for inclusion in your nutritional plan. Legumes are high in protein and fiber and low in fat. Legumes include dry beans and peas like kidney, navy, and pinto beans, chickpeas, split peas, and lentils.

**Key Recommendation**: Legumes may also count as a protein or vegetable.

## Recommendations:

- Enjoy pinto and kidney beans on a salad
- Try a split pea or lentil soup
- Add legumes to salads and casseroles

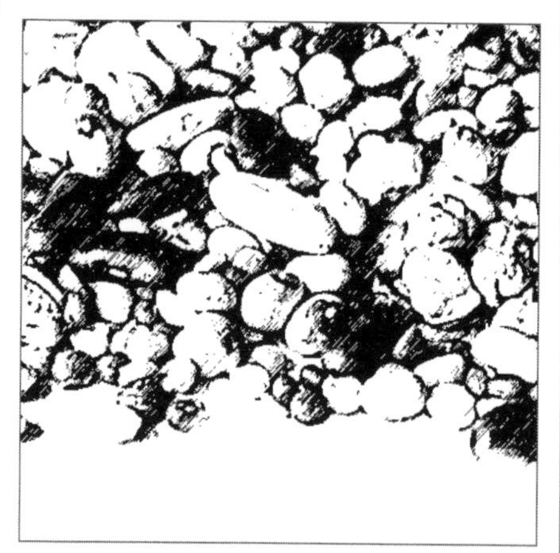

**Legumes**

| Calories per ½ Cup "cooked" | Dry Beans and Peas and Lentils |
|---|---|
| 90 | Black-Eyed Peas |
| 103 | Red Beans |
| 104 | Split Peas |
| 106 | Kidney Beans |
| 106 | Great Northern Beans |
| 107 | Lima Beans |
| 109 | Black Beans |
| 110 | Pinto Beans |
| 113 | Lentils |
| 125 | Small White Beans |
| 137 | Garbanzo Beans |
| 151 | Soybeans |

# Nuts & Seeds

Nuts and seeds are also considered part of the protein food group but as with legumes are listed here separately to draw attention to their important health benefits and the need for inclusion in your nutritional plan. They contain healthy fats that have been shown to decrease the risk of heart disease, cancer, and other chronic diseases.

**Key Recommendation**: Nuts and seeds may also count as a protein.

## Recommendations:

- Choose nuts as a snack
- Place nuts on salads and in main dishes
- Use pine nuts in peso sauce for pasta
- Add slivered almonds to steamed vegetables
- Add toasted peanuts to stir fry instead of meat
- Sprinkle a few chopped up nuts on low fat ice cream or frozen yogurt
- Add walnuts or pecans to green salad

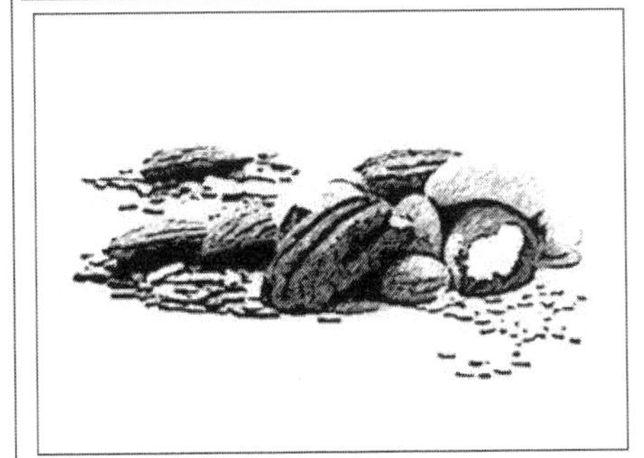

| Nuts & Seeds | |
|---|---|
| Calories per ½ Ounce | Nuts and Seeds |
| (1 Tbl. seeds) (2 Tbl. Nuts) | |
| 37 | Flaxseed (whole) |
| 40 | Flaxseed (ground) |
| 52 | Sesame Seeds |
| 63 | Pumpkin Seeds |
| 78 | Cashews |
| 81 | Pistachios |
| 82 | Almonds |
| 83 | Peanuts |
| 83 | Sunflower Seeds |
| 89 | Hazelnuts |
| 93 | Walnuts |
| 95 | Pine Nuts |
| 95 | Brazil Nuts |
| 98 | Pecans |
| 100 | Macadamia |
| | |
| | |
| | |
| | |

# Fats/Oils & Condiments

High quality fats like monounsaturated fats and Omega-3 fatty acids promote health. Saturated fats hydrogenated fats, and trans fats increase the risk of disease and should be significantly limited in one's diet or eliminated.

**Key Recommendation**: Choose healthy fats and low calorie sugar based products.

## Recommendations:

- Use olive oil when cooking
- Add flaxseed to salads and casseroles
- Avoid all trans fats
- Reduce the amount of fat/oil used in baking or substitute with applesauce
- Consider low calorie sugar based products
- Choose light margarines, mayonnaise, and salad dressings
- Try salsa in place of high fat dips

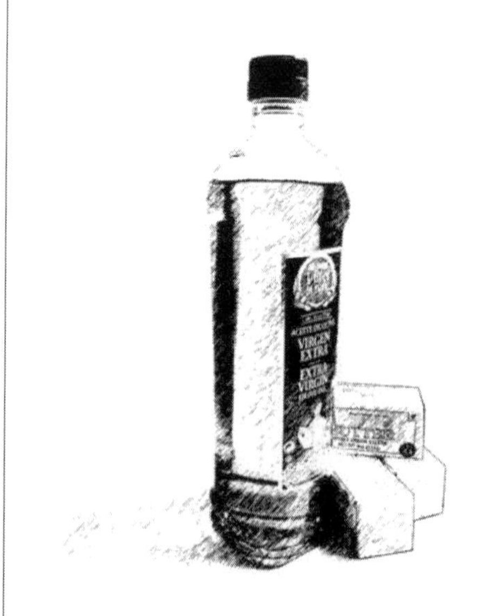

| Fats/Oils & Condiments | |
|---|---|
| Calories per Tablespoon | Fats/Oils & Condiments |
| 2 | Vinegar |
| 5 | Salsa |
| 10 | Fat-Free Mayonnaise |
| 12 | Mustard |
| 13 | Sour Cream (non fat) |
| 16 | Ketchup |
| 25 | Whipped Cream |
| 26 | Gravy |
| 30 | Coconut (shredded) |
| 30 | Salad Dressing (light) |
| 35 | Barbeque Sauce |
| 50 | Jam/Jelly |
| 50 | Margarine (light) |
| 50 | Mayonnaise (light) |
| 50 | Sugar |
| 58 | Syrup |
| 60 | Hot Fudge |
| 65 | Honey |
| 75 | Salad Dressing |
| 95 | Peanut Butter |
| 100 | Butter |
| 100 | Margarine |
| 100 | Mayonnaise |
| 120 | Oils (all) |

## How to Read a Nutrition Food Label
### Source: U.S. Food and Drug Administration

Certainly the best source of calorie information for a food is its Nutritional Food Label. Those successful at weight management know the "ins" and "outs" of reading a Nutritional Food Label and use it to accurately determine the number of calories they will consume in a serving of the product. Learning this skill is part of your behavioral change process and an integral element for your success, as well as a fun and informative activity at the grocery store. As you learn its components and apply it in shopping for and evaluating foods, your nutritional wisdom will grow and you become more empowered to ***act*** effectively in the selection of leaner and healthier foods.

**Nutrition Facts**

Serving Size 1 cup (228g)
Servings Per Container about 2

**Amount Per Serving**

| **Calories** 250 | Calories from Fat 110 |
|---|---|
| | **% Daily Value*** |
| **Total Fat** 12g | **18%** |
| Saturated Fat 3g | **15%** |
| *Trans* Fat 3g | |
| **Cholesterol** 30mg | **10%** |
| **Sodium** 470mg | **20%** |
| **Total Carbohydrate** 31g | **10%** |
| Dietary Fiber 0g | 0% |
| Sugars 5g | |
| **Proteins** 5g | |
| Vitamin A | 4% |
| Vitamin C | 2% |
| Calcium | 20% |
| Iron | 4% |

* Percent Daily Values are based on a 2,000 calorie diet. Your Daily Values may be higher or lower depending on your calorie needs:

| | Calories: | 2,000 | 2,500 |
|---|---|---|---|
| Total Fat | Less than | 65g | 80g |
| Saturated Fat | | Less than | 20g |
| 25g | | | |
| Cholesterol | Less than | 300mg | 300mg |
| Sodium | Less than | 2,400mg | 2,400mg |
| Total Carbohydrate | | 300g | 375g |

For educational purposes only. This label does not meet the labeling requirements described in 21 CFR 101.9.

**1 Serving Size**

This section is the basis for determining number of calories, amount of each nutrient, and %DVs of a food. Use it to compare a serving size to how much you actually eat. Serving sizes are given in familiar units, such as cups or pieces, followed by the metric amount, e.g., number of grams.

**2 Amount of Calories**

If you want to manage your weight (lose, gain, or maintain), this section is especially helpful. The amount of calories is listed on the left side. The right side shows how many calories in one serving come from fat. In this example, there are 250 calories, 110 of which come from fat. The key is to balance how many calories you eat with how many calories your body uses. ***Tip:*** *Remember that a product that's fat-free isn't necessarily calorie-free.*

**3 Limit these Nutrients**

Eating too much total fat (including saturated fat and trans fat), cholesterol, or sodium may increase your risk of certain chronic diseases, such as heart disease, some cancers, or high blood pressure. The goal is to stay below 100%DV for each of these nutrients per day.

**4 Get Enough of these Nutrients**

Americans often don't get enough dietary fiber, vitamin A, vitamin C, calcium, and iron in their diets. Eating enough of these nutrients may improve your health and help reduce the risk of some diseases and conditions.

**5 Percent (%) Daily Value**

This section tells you whether the nutrients (total fat, sodium, dietary fiber, etc.) in one serving of food contribute a little or a lot to your total daily diet.

The %DVs are based on a 2,000-calorie diet. Each listed nutrient is based on 100% of the recommended amounts for that nutrient. For example, 18% for total fat means that one serving furnishes 18% of the total amount of fat that you could eat in a day and stay within public health recommendations. Use the Quick Guide to Percent DV (%DV): 5%DV or less is low and 20%DV or more is high.

**6 Footnote with Daily Values (DVs)**

The footnote provides information about the DVs for important nutrients, including fats, sodium and fiber. The DVs are listed for people who eat 2,000 or 2,500 calories each day.

- The amounts for total fat, saturated fat, cholesterol, and sodium are maximum amounts. That means you should try to stay below the amounts listed.

# Step 6

# Become An Expert in the Use of Your Daily Nutrition & Activity Record and Weekly Reflection Form

As has been previously stated, in order to effectively manage body weight you must know how many calories you consume in a day in comparison to the number of calories you burn. The difference between these two amounts represents the resulting weight loss that you should expect simply based on the math. Granted, sometimes weight loss plateaus or a less than expected weight loss amount that you may experience during the course of your journey may seem to challenge the math. However, your consistent consumption of fewer calories compared to the amount you burn will lead to the desired weight loss as your body conforms to the negative energy balance.

The **Daily Nutrition & Activity Record** is where you record the essential information specific to the calories you consume in food and drink and the calories you expend through exercise. Your accurate and consistent completion of this form each day will have a profound impact on your success. To maximize its usefulness:

1. Record your specific goal or action for the day. Ask yourself, what new, achievable, and meaningful quest do you want to focus on and be mindful of for that day?

**Nutritional Information**

2. Record the specific foods and beverages consumed throughout the day *at the time you consume them*. Be mindful to *plan ahead* what you will eat that day and execute your food and beverage intake to stay within your nutritional plan calorie level. Also, strive to consume the food group recommendations as best you can to ensure balanced, health promoting nutrition.
3. Record the amount and associated calories of the foods and beverages consumed.

> Note: There are a variety of resources from which to obtain the calorie value of a food or beverage. There are the pages in this booklet, certain APPs, online data bases, some restaurant menus, and of course the Nutrition Food Label on most products. Research has shown that for long-term success in weight management a person should actually learn the calorie value of foods commonly eaten. That learning process is best achieved when the individual actually records/writes down what they consumed and the calorie amounts. Yes, this can take some effort and at times can be somewhat tedious, but it is part of the behavioral change process and the becoming of a new and more knowledgeable person who can then exercise wisdom in all future nutritional decision making. The right mindset is to look forward to enjoying the opportunity to learn by recording the information; making a game of this acquisition of new knowledge.

4. Check off the boxes of the respective food group servings as you consume them as well as a water drop symbol each time you drink 8 ounces of water or a calorie free drink. Remember, the better you get at consuming the recommended servings for each of the food groups (while remaining at your target calorie level) the better the disease protecting nutrition you are obtaining.
5. At the end of each day, total and record the calories consumed for the day.

**Physical Activity Information**

6. Record the total number of calories expended in planned exercise for the day.

> The chart for calculating energy expenditure during selected exercises is located on page 22 of this book. In addition, certain exercise machines can estimate calorie burn during their use based on your body weight that is entered into the machine. An accurate recording of the calories you burn through exercise is vital in the calculation of projected weight loss.
>
> The National Institutes of Health (NIH) and the American College of Sports Medicine (ACSM) guidelines for weight loss and weight loss maintenance recommend at least 60 minutes of daily exercise to burn additional calories toward increasing the negative energy balance for weight loss. Because the 60 minutes can be acquired in 10 minute increments, six boxes each representing 10 minutes of exercise are provided for you to mark off when 10 minutes of exercise has been completed.

7. Check off the appropriate box indicating if you completed resistance training that targeted the 1) upper body, 2) lower body, and/or 3) body core. Remember, resistance training is vital to helping maintain lean body mass during weight loss efforts as well as your metabolic rate.

The **Weekly Reflection Form** is basically your week in review. It is where you record the totals for the week in both calories consumed in food and beverages and calories expended in planned exercise. Because calories are also burned to support your metabolism (resting metabolic rate) and activities of daily living, these values will also need to be factored into the equation. To obtain the needed information to work the "Calculation for Projected Weight Loss for the Week":

1. Record the total calories consumed for each day of the previous week then total the amount and place that figure in the "Total Calories Consumed" box of the equation.
2. Determine the total calories burned in supporting your resting metabolic needs of a day as well as those calories burned to support your activities of daily living. This information is found in "Step 5" of this book on page 33. Simply take the amount listed and multiply it by 7 to account for all days of the week.
3. Record the total calories burned from planned exercise for each day of the previous week and then total the amount and place that figure in the "Total Exercise Calories Burned" box of the equation.
4. Now work the equation by subtracting the "Activities of Daily Living" and the "Total Exercise Calories Burned" values from the "Total Calories Consumed" amount. This represents the "Calorie Difference" between calorie intake and expenditure. Finally, divide that amount by 3,500 (the number of calories in one pound of body fat) to determine the "Projected Weight Loss" amount in pounds.
5. In the "My Wellness Journal" section record your thoughts, feelings, any questions you may have, or anything you learned that week that you feel will benefit your efforts as you move forward on your journey of change and becoming. Also record a positive/constructive thought about you or your efforts. You are acting in an independent and empowered way; acknowledge your efforts in a positive statement of self.

Week 1

## Daily Nutrition & Activity Record

Mon Tue Wed (Thu) Fri Sat Sun — Date: Jan 9

Goal or Action for the Day:

| Food & Beverage | Amount Vol. Wt/# | Calories |
|---|---|---|
| Cooked oatmeal | 1 cup | 166 |
| Blueberries | ½ cup | 42 |
| 1% milk | [illegible] | [illegible] |
| | Total | 1606 |

### # of Servings by Calorie Level

| | | | 1200 | 1400 | 1600 | 1800 | 2000 | 2200 | 2400 |
|---|---|---|---|---|---|---|---|---|---|
| Grains | ☒ | ☒ | ☒ | +☒ | +☒ | +☒ | +☐ | +☐ | +☐ +☐ |
| Fruits | | ☒ | ☒ | | | +☐ | | | |
| Veggies | ☒ | ☒ | ☒ | | +☐ | | +☐ | | +☐ |
| Dairy | ☒ | ☒ | ☒ | | | | | | |
| Protein | ☒ ☒ | ☒ | ☒ | | +☐ | | | | +☐ |
| Fats/Oils | | ☒ | ☐ | | | +☐ | | | |

Legumes: ■ 1200-1800; ☐ 2000-2400

Nuts & Seeds: ■ 1200; ☒ 1400-2000; ☐☐ 2200-2400

Water: ☒☒☒☒☒☒OO–OOOO

**Physical Activity**

Total Calories Burned: 310

Time (10 min. increments): ☒10 ☒10 ☒10

Resistance Training: Upper ☒ Core ☐ Lower ☐

## Weekly Reflection Form

Week 1

Date: | Weight:

| Nutritional Summary | | | Physical Activity Summary | | |
|---|---|---|---|---|---|
| Day of Week | Calories Consumed | # Fruits & Vegs | Day of Week | Calories Burned | Time in minutes |
| Monday | 1641 | | Monday | 310 | |
| Tuesday | 1588 | | Tuesday | 452 | |
| Wednesday | 1612 | | Wednesday | 320 | |
| Thursday | 1627 | | Thursday | 460 | |
| Friday | 1648 | | Friday | 320 | |
| Saturday | 1566 | | Saturday | 517 | |
| Sunday | 1710 | | Sunday | 0 | |
| Total | 11,392 | | Total | 2,379 | |

### Calculation for Projected Weight loss for the Week

| Total Calories Consumed | | ADL: (RMRx1.25x7) | | Total Exercise Cals Burned | | Calorie Difference | | Calories in 1 pound fat | | Projected Weight Loss | |
|---|---|---|---|---|---|---|---|---|---|---|---|
| 11,392 | - | 14,787 | - | 2,379 | = | -5,774 | ÷ | 3,500 | = | -1.65 | lbs. |

My Wellness Journal - Thoughts / Feelings / Questions:

Week 1

# Daily Nutrition & Activity Record

Mon Tue **Wed** Thu Fri Sat Sun — Date: 1/28

Goal or Action for the Day: eat planned meals

| Food & Beverage | Amount (Vol. Wt/#) | Calories |
|---|---|---|
| oatmeal - homemade | 1/2 c. | 75 |
| flax seed | 1 T | 55 |
| adams peanut butter | 1 T | 105 |
| blueberries | 1/2 c. | 40 |
| | | |
| almonds | 18 | 123 |
| kind granola bar | 1 | 150 |
| hard boiled egg | 1 | 78 |
| carrots - baby | 10 | 35 |
| banana | 1/2 | 90 |
| | | |
| almond milk | 2 c. | 60 |
| protein powder | 1 scoop | 140 |
| dark chocolate | 2 pieces | 84 |
| | | |
| lettuce | 1 cup | 7 |
| nut thin crackers | 16 | 130 |
| dressing | 2 T | 70 |
| tuna | 1 can | 90 |
| **Total** | | 1332 |

## # of Servings by Calorie Level

1200 1400 1600 1800 2000 2200 2400

Grains
Fruits
Veggies
Dairy
Protein
Fats/Oils

Legumes: 1200-1800; 2000-2400

Nuts & Seeds: 1200; 1400-2000; 2200-2400

Water

## Physical Activity

Total Calories Burned: ~500

Time (10 min. increments): 10 10 10 10 10 10

Resistance Training: Upper Core Lower

# Daily Nutrition & Activity Record

Mon Tue Wed (Thu) Fri Sat Sun — Date: 1/29

Goal or Action for the Day: usually don't exercise, do it!

| Food & Beverage | Amount (Vol. Wt/#) | Calories |
|---|---|---|
| oatmeal - homemade | 1/2 c | 75 |
| flax seed | 1T | 55 |
| peanut butter | 1T | 105 |
| blueberries | 1/2 c. | 40 |
| | | |
| almonds | 18 | 123 |
| kind granola bar | 1 | 150 |
| hard boiled egg | 1 | 78 |
| carrots - baby | 10 | 35 |
| apple | 1 | 90 |
| | | |
| almond milk | 2 c | 60 |
| protein powder | 1sc. | 190 |
| | | |
| lettuce | 1 c. | 7 |
| nut thins crackers | 16 | 130 |
| dressing | 2T | 70 |
| tuna | 1 can | 90 |
| dark chocolate | 2 pieces | 84 |
| Total | | 1332 |

## # of Servings by Calorie Level

1200 1400 1600 1800 2000 2200 2400

Grains
Fruits
Veggies
Dairy
Protein
Fats/Oils

Legumes: 1200-1800; 2000-2400

Nuts & Seeds: 1200; 1400-2000; 2200-2400

Water

## Physical Activity

Total Calories Burned: ~400

Time (10 min. increments): 10 10 10 10 10 10

Resistance Training: Upper Core Lower



Week 1

Week 1

# Daily Nutrition & Activity Record

Mon Tue Wed Thu (Fri) Sat Sun

Date: 1/30

Goal or Action for the Day: eat healthy

| Food & Beverage | Amount Vol. Wt/# | Calories |
|---|---|---|
| oatmeal - home made | 1/2c. | 75 |
| flax seeds | 1T | 55 |
| adams peanut butter | 1T | 105 |
| tropical fruit | 1/2c. | 50 |
| | | |
| almonds | 18 | 123 |
| kind granola bar | 1 | 150 |
| carrots - baby | 10 | 35 |
| banana | 1 | 90 |
| | | |
| almond milk | 2c. | 60 |
| 1 scoop protein powder | 1 | 140 |
| hard boiled egg | 1 | 78 |
| | | |
| gator jacks sandwich | 1 | 300 |
| cookie | 1 | 200 |
| dark chocolate | 2p. | 84 |
| Total | | 1545 |

## # of Servings by Calorie Level

| | | | 1200 | 1400 | 1600 | 1800 | 2000 | 2200 | 2400 |
|---|---|---|---|---|---|---|---|---|---|
| Grains | ☑ | ☑ | ☑ | + ☐ ☐ | + ☐ | + ☐ | + ☐ | + ☐ | + ☐ |
| Fruits | | ☑ | ☑ | | | + ☐ | | | |
| Veggies | ☑ | ☑ | ☐ | | + ☐ | | + ☐ | | + ☐ |
| Dairy | ☑ | ☑ | ☑ | | | | | | |
| Protein | ☑ ☑ | ☑ | ☑ | | + ☐ | | | | + ☐ |
| Fats/Oils | | ☑ | ☑ | | | + ☐ | | | |

Legumes: ◩ 1200-1800; ☐ 2000-2400

Nuts & Seeds: ◩ 1200; ☐ 1400-2000; ☐ ☐ 2200-2400

Water (drops, 8 of 12 marked)

**Physical Activity**

Total Calories Burned: ~200

Time (10 min. increments)

| 10 (✓) | 10 (✓) | 10 (✓) |
|---|---|---|
| 10 (✓) | 10 | 10 |

Resistance Training

Upper ☐ Core ☒ Lower ☒

# Daily Nutrition & Activity Record

Week 1

Mon Tue Wed Thu Fri (Sat) Sun

Date: 1/31

Goal or Action for the Day: fast...

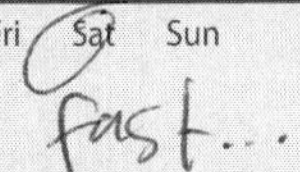

| Food & Beverage | Amount Vol. Wt/# | Calories |
|---|---|---|
| 3 eggs | 3 | 230 |
| turkey bacon | 2 | 115 |
| | | |
| kind granola bar | 1 | 150 |
| banana | 1 | 90 |
| chocolate milk (almond) | 1 c. | 100 |
| | | |
| Salad @ Hickory - chicken | 1 | 500 |
| Ice cream | 1 cup | 300 |

Total 1485

## # of Servings by Calorie Level

| | 1200 | 1400 | 1600 | 1800 | 2000 | 2200 | 2400 |
|---|---|---|---|---|---|---|---|
| Grains | ☐ ☐ ☐ | +☐ ☐ | +☐ | +☐ | +☐ | +☐ | +☐ |
| Fruits | ☑ ☐ | | | +☐ | | | |
| Veggies | ☑ ☑ ☑ | | +☐ | | +☐ | | +☐ |
| Dairy | ☑ ☑ ☐ | | | | | | |
| Protein | ☑ ☑ ☑ ☑ | | +☐ | | | | +☐ |
| Fats/Oils | ☐ ☐ | | | +☐ | | | |

Legumes: ◪ 1200-1800; ☐ 2000-2400

Nuts & Seeds: ◪ 1200; ☐ 1400-2000; ☐ ☐ 2200-2400

Water: 💧💧💧💧💧💧💧💧 💧💧💧💧 (crossed out)

## Physical Activity

Total Calories Burned: ~ 100

Time (10 min. increments)

| 10 (crossed) | 10 (crossed) | 10 (crossed) |
|---|---|---|
| 10 | 10 | 10 |

Resistance Training

| Upper | Core | Lower |
|---|---|---|
| ☐ | ☒ | ☐ |

Week 1

# Daily Nutrition & Activity Record

Mon Tue Wed Thu Fri Sat Sun (circled) Date: 2/1

Goal or Action for the Day: break fast! eat good.

| Food & Beverage | Amount (Vol. Wt/#) | Calories |
|---|---|---|
| chips | 20-Chip | 150 |
| homemade salsa chunky | 1c. | 60 |
| apple | 1 | 95 |
| brownies | 2 | 250 |
| lasagna w/ veggies | 1 | 180 |
| dark chocolate | 2p. | 84 |
| | Total | 819 |

## # of Servings by Calorie Level

| | | | 1200 | | 1400 | 1600 | 1800 | 2000 | 2200 | 2400 |
|---|---|---|---|---|---|---|---|---|---|---|
| Grains | ☑ | ☑ | ☐ | +☐ | ☐ | +☐ | +☐ | +☐ | +☐ | +☐ |
| Fruits | | ☑ | ☐ | | | | +☐ | | | |
| Veggies | ☑ | ☑ | ☑ | | | +☐ | | +☐ | | +☐ |
| Dairy | ☑ | ☐ | ☐ | | | | | | | |
| Protein ☑ | ☐ | ☐ | ☐ | | | +☐ | | | | +☐ |
| Fats/Oils | | ☑ | ☐ | | | | +☐ | | | |

Legumes: ◪ 1200-1800; ☐ 2000-2400

Nuts & Seeds: ◪ 1200; ☐ 1400-2000; ☐ ☐ 2200-2400

Water (crossed out)

**Physical Activity**

Total Calories Burned: (crossed out)

Time (10 min. increments): 10 10 10 10 10 10

Resistance Training: Upper ☐ Core ☐ Lower ☐

# Daily Nutrition & Activity Record

Week 1

Mon Tue Wed Thu Fri Sat Sun (Mon circled)

Date: 2/2

Goal or Action for the Day: more veggies

| Food & Beverage | Amount Vol. Wt/# | Calories |
|---|---|---|
| oatmeal - homemade | 1/2 c. | 75 |
| flax seeds | 1 T | 55 |
| peanut butter | 1 T | 105 |
| tropical fruit | 1/2 c. | 50 |
| | | |
| 1 kind bar | 1 | 150 |
| 18 almonds | 18 | 123 |
| dark chocolate | 2 | 84 |
| hard boiled eggs | 1 | 78 |
| 10 carrots | 10 | 35 |
| apple | 1 | 95 |
| | | |
| 1 scoop protein powder | 1 | 140 |
| almond milk (1 choc, 1 reg) | 2 c. | 80 |
| | | |
| lettuce | 1 c. | 7 |
| nut thins | 16 | 130 |
| dressing | 2 T | 70 |
| tuna | 1 can | 90 |
| | Total | 1350 |

## # of Servings by Calorie Level

1200 1400 1600 1800 2000 2200 2400

Grains
Fruits
Veggies
Dairy
Protein
Fats/Oils

Legumes: 1200-1800; 2000-2400

Nuts & Seeds: 1200; 1400-2000; 2200-2400

Water

## Physical Activity

Total Calories Burned: ~500

Time (10 min. increments): 10 10 10 10 10 10

Resistance Training: Upper Core Lower

Week 1

# Daily Nutrition & Activity Record

Mon (Tue) Wed Thu Fri Sat Sun    Date: 2/3

Goal or Action for the Day: workout!

| Food & Beverage | Amount Vol. Wt/# | Calories |
|---|---|---|
| oatmeal - home made | 1/2 c. | 75 |
| flax seeds | 1 T | 55 |
| peanut butter | 1 T | 105 |
| blue berries | 1/2 c. | 40 |
| | | |
| kind bar | 1 | 150 |
| carrots | 10 | 35 |
| almonds | 18 | 123 |
| dark chocolate | 2 p. | 84 |
| apple | 1 | 95 |
| | | |
| almond milk | 2 c. | 60 |
| protein powder | 1 s. | 140 |
| | | |
| subway | 1 6 in. | 260 |
| dark chocolate | 2 p. | 84 |
| | Total | 1306 |

## # of Servings by Calorie Level

| | 1200 | 1400 | 1600 | 1800 | 2000 | 2200 | 2400 |
|---|---|---|---|---|---|---|---|
| Grains | ☑ ☑ ☑ | + ☐ | ☐ + ☐ | + ☐ | + ☐ | + ☐ | + ☐ |
| Fruits | ☑ ☑ | | | + ☐ | | | |
| Veggies | ☑ ☑ ☑ | | + ☐ | | + ☐ | | + ☐ |
| Dairy | ☑ ☑ ☐ | | | | | | |
| Protein | ☑ ☑ ☑ ☑ | | + ☐ | | | | + ☐ |
| Fats/Oils | ☑ ☑ | | | + ☐ | | | |

Legumes: 1200-1800; 2000-2400

Nuts & Seeds: 1200; 1400-2000; 2200-2400

Water

**Physical Activity**

Total Calories Burned: ~300

Time (10 min. increments): 10 10 10 10 10 10

Resistance Training: Upper Core Lower

# Weekly Reflection Form

Week 1

| Date: 2/4 | Weight: 147 |
|---|---|

| Nutritional Summary | | | Physical Activity Summary | | |
|---|---|---|---|---|---|
| Day of Week | Calories Consumed | # Fruits & Vegs | Day of Week | Calories Burned | Time in minutes |
| Monday | 1350 | 4 | Monday | 500 | 60 |
| Tuesday | 1306 | 5 | Tuesday | 300 | 50 |
| Wednesday | 1332 | 4 | Wednesday | 500 | 60 |
| Thursday | 1332 | 4 | Thursday | 400 | 50 |
| Friday | 1545 | 4 | Friday | 200 | 40 |
| Saturday | 1485 | 3 | Saturday | 100 | 30 |
| Sunday | 819 | 4 | Sunday | — | |
| Total | 9169 | 28 | Total | 2000 | 290 |

## Calculation for Projected Weight loss for the Week

| Total Calories Consumed | | ADL: (RMRx1.25x7) | | Total Exercise Cals Burned | | Calorie Difference | | Calories in 1 pound fat | | Projected Weight Loss |
|---|---|---|---|---|---|---|---|---|---|---|
| 9169 | - | 12810 | - | 2000 | = | -5641 | ÷ | 3,500 | = | -1.6 lbs. |

**My Wellness Journal - Thoughts / Feelings / Questions:**

Went well. I ate really good I thought. The weekends are harder for me to have the structure I usually do in the week days, but overall it went great.
My workouts were kind of all over the place - usually their here consistent, and usually I eat more, especially on sunday & if I go home for dinner.

**Your Positive & Constructive Statement About Self:**

I was surprised! it wasn't so bad. I did pretty well.

Week 2

# Daily Nutrition & Activity Record

Mon Tue Wed Thu Fri Sat Sun Date:

Goal or Action for the Day:

| Food & Beverage | Amount Vol. Wt/# | Calories |
|---|---|---|
| | | |
| | | |
| | | |
| | | |
| | | |
| | | |
| | | |
| | | |
| | | |
| | | |
| | | |
| | | |
| | | |
| | | |
| | | |
| | | |
| | | |
| | | |
| | | |
| | | |
| | | |
| | | |
| | | |
| | | |
| | | |
| | | |
| | Total | |

**# of Servings by Calorie Level**

1200 1400 1600 1800 2000 2200 2400

Grains

Fruits

Veggies

Dairy

Protein

Fats/Oils

Legumes 1200-1800 2000-2400

Nuts & Seeds 1200 1400-2000 2200-2400

Water

**Physical Activity**

Total Calories Burned

Time (10 min. increments)

| 10 | 10 | 10 |
|---|---|---|
| 10 | 10 | 10 |

Resistance Training

Upper Core Lower

# Daily Nutrition & Activity Record

Mon Tue Wed Thu Fri Sat Sun Date:

Goal or Action for the Day:

| Food & Beverage | Amount Vol. Wt/# | Calories |
|---|---|---|
| | | |
| | Total | |

## # of Servings by Calorie Level

1200 1400 1600 1800 2000 2200 2400

Grains

Fruits

Veggies

Dairy

Protein

Fats/Oils

Legumes 1200-1800 2000-2400

Nuts & Seeds 1200 1400-2000 2200-2400

Water

**Physical Activity**

Total Calories Burned

Time (10 min. increments)

| 10 | 10 | 10 |
|---|---|---|
| 10 | 10 | 10 |

Resistance Training

Upper Core Lower

Week 2

Week 2

# Daily Nutrition & Activity Record

Mon Tue Wed Thu Fri Sat Sun Date:

Goal or Action for the Day:

| Food & Beverage | Amount Vol. Wt/# | Calories |
|---|---|---|
| | | |
| | | |
| | | |
| | | |
| | | |
| | | |
| | | |
| | | |
| | | |
| | | |
| | | |
| | | |
| | | |
| | | |
| | | |
| | | |
| | | |
| | | |
| | | |
| | | |
| | | |
| | | |
| | | |
| | | |
| | | |
| | Total | |

## # of Servings by Calorie Level

1200 1400 1600 1800 2000 2200 2400

Grains

Fruits

Veggies

Dairy

Protein

Fats/Oils

Legumes 1200-1800 / 2000-2400

Nuts & Seeds 1200 / 1400-2000 / 2200-2400

Water

**Physical Activity**

Total Calories Burned

Time (10 min. increments)

| 10 | 10 | 10 |
|---|---|---|
| 10 | 10 | 10 |

Resistance Training

Upper Core Lower

# Daily Nutrition & Activity Record

Mon Tue Wed Thu Fri Sat Sun Date:

Goal or Action for the Day:

| Food & Beverage | Amount Vol. Wt/# | Calories |
|---|---|---|
| | | |
| | Total | |

Week 2

## # of Servings by Calorie Level

| | | | 1200 | | 1400 | 1600 | 1800 | 2000 | 2200 | 2400 |
|---|---|---|---|---|---|---|---|---|---|---|
| Grains | ☐ | ☐ | ☐ | +☐ | ☐ | +☐ | +☐ | +☐ | +☐ | +☐ |
| Fruits | | ☐ | ☐ | | | | +☐ | | | |
| Veggies | ☐ | ☐ | ☐ | | | +☐ | | +☐ | | +☐ |
| Dairy | ☐ | ☐ | ☐ | | | | | | | |
| Protein ☐ | ☐ | ☐ | ☐ | | | +☐ | | | | +☐ |
| Fats/Oils | | ☐ | ☐ | | | | +☐ | | | |

Legumes ◩ 1200-1800 ☐ 2000-2400

Nuts & Seeds ◩ 1200 ☐ 1400-2000 ☐☐ 2200-2400

Water 💧💧💧💧💧💧💧–💧💧💧💧

**Physical Activity**

Total Calories Burned

Time (10 min. increments)

| 10 | 10 | 10 |
|---|---|---|
| 10 | 10 | 10 |

Resistance Training

Upper ☐ Core ☐ Lower ☐

Week 2

# Daily Nutrition & Activity Record

Mon Tue Wed Thu Fri Sat Sun Date:

Goal or Action for the Day:

| Food & Beverage | Amount Vol. Wt/# | Calories |
|---|---|---|
| | | |
| | Total | |

## # of Servings by Calorie Level

1200 1400 1600 1800 2000 2200 2400

Grains

Fruits

Veggies

Dairy

Protein

Fats/Oils

Legumes 1200-1800 2000-2400

Nuts & Seeds 1200 1400-2000 2200-2400

Water

**Physical Activity**

Total Calories Burned

Time (10 min. increments)

10 10 10
10 10 10

Resistance Training

Upper Core Lower

# Daily Nutrition & Activity Record

Mon Tue Wed Thu Fri Sat Sun Date:

Goal or Action for the Day:

| Food & Beverage | Amount Vol. Wt/# | Calories |
|---|---|---|
| | | |
| | Total | |

Week 2

## # of Servings by Calorie Level

| | | | 1200 | | 1400 | 1600 | 1800 | 2000 | 2200 | 2400 |
|---|---|---|---|---|---|---|---|---|---|---|
| Grains | ☐ | ☐ | ☐ | +☐ | ☐ | +☐ | +☐ | +☐ | +☐ | +☐ |
| Fruits | | ☐ | ☐ | | | | +☐ | | | |
| Veggies | ☐ | ☐ | ☐ | | | +☐ | | +☐ | | +☐ |
| Dairy | ☐ | ☐ | ☐ | | | | | | | |
| Protein ☐ | ☐ | ☐ | ☐ | | | +☐ | | | | +☐ |
| Fats/Oils | | ☐ | ☐ | | | | +☐ | | | |

Legumes ◪ 1200-1800
☐ 2000-2400

Nuts & Seeds ◪ 1200
☐ 1400-2000
☐☐ 2200-2400

Water 💧💧💧💧💧💧💧💧–💧💧💧💧

**Physical Activity**

Total Calories Burned

Time (10 min. increments)

| 10 | 10 | 10 |
|---|---|---|
| 10 | 10 | 10 |

Resistance Training

Upper ☐ Core ☐ Lower ☐

# Daily Nutrition & Activity Record

Mon Tue Wed Thu Fri Sat Sun Date:

Goal or Action for the Day:

| Food & Beverage | Amount Vol. Wt/# | Calories |
|---|---|---|
| | | |
| | | |
| | | |
| | | |
| | | |
| | | |
| | | |
| | | |
| | | |
| | | |
| | | |
| | | |
| | | |
| | | |
| | | |
| | | |
| | | |
| | | |
| | | |
| | | |
| | | |
| | | |
| | | |
| | | |
| | | |
| | | |
| | Total | |

Week 2

## # of Servings by Calorie Level

| | 1200 | 1400 | 1600 | 1800 | 2000 | 2200 | 2400 |
|---|---|---|---|---|---|---|---|
| Grains | ☐ ☐ ☐ | + ☐ | ☐ + ☐ | + ☐ | + ☐ | + ☐ | + ☐ |
| Fruits | ☐ ☐ | | | + ☐ | | | |
| Veggies | ☐ ☐ ☐ | | + ☐ | | + ☐ | | + ☐ |
| Dairy | ☐ ☐ ☐ | | | | | | |
| Protein | ☐ ☐ ☐ ☐ | | + ☐ | | | | + ☐ |
| Fats/Oils | ☐ ☐ | | | + ☐ | | | |

Legumes ◪ 1200-1800 ☐ 2000-2400

Nuts & Seeds ◪ 1200 ☐ 1400-2000 ☐ ☐ 2200-2400

Water 💧💧💧💧💧💧💧💧 – 💧💧💧💧

**Physical Activity**

Total Calories Burned

Time (10 min. increments)

| 10 | 10 | 10 |
|---|---|---|
| 10 | 10 | 10 |

Resistance Training

Upper ☐ Core ☐ Lower ☐

# Weekly Reflection Form

| Date: | Weight: |
|---|---|

| **Nutritional Summary** | | | **Physical Activity Summary** | | |
|---|---|---|---|---|---|
| Day of Week | Calories Consumed | # Fruits & Vegs | Day of Week | Calories Burned | Time in minutes |
| Monday | | | Monday | | |
| Tuesday | | | Tuesday | | |
| Wednesday | | | Wednesday | | |
| Thursday | | | Thursday | | |
| Friday | | | Friday | | |
| Saturday | | | Saturday | | |
| Sunday | | | Sunday | | |
| Total | | | Total | | |

**Calculation for Projected Weight loss for the Week**

| Total Calories Consumed | ADL: (RMRx1.25x7) | Total Exercise Cals Burned | Calorie Difference | Calories in 1 pound fat | Projected Weight Loss |
|---|---|---|---|---|---|
| ________ - | ________ - | ________ = | ________ | ÷ 3,500 = | ________ lbs. |

**My Wellness Journal - Thoughts / Feelings / Questions:**

**Your Positive & Constructive Statement About Self:**

Week 2

# Daily Nutrition & Activity Record

Mon Tue Wed Thu Fri Sat Sun Date:

Goal or Action for the Day:

| Food & Beverage | Amount Vol. Wt/# | Calories |
|---|---|---|
| | | |
| | Total | |

## # of Servings by Calorie Level

| | | | | 1200 | | 1400 | 1600 | 1800 | 2000 | 2200 | 2400 |
|---|---|---|---|---|---|---|---|---|---|---|---|
| Grains | | ☐ | ☐ | ☐ | +☐ | ☐ | +☐ | +☐ | +☐ | +☐ | +☐ |
| Fruits | | | ☐ | ☐ | | | | +☐ | | | |
| Veggies | | ☐ | ☐ | ☐ | | | +☐ | | +☐ | | +☐ |
| Dairy | | ☐ | ☐ | ☐ | | | | | | | |
| Protein | ☐ | ☐ | ☐ | ☐ | | | +☐ | | | | +☐ |
| Fats/Oils | | | ☐ | ☐ | | | | +☐ | | | |

Legumes ◪ 1200-1800 ☐ 2000-2400

Nuts & Seeds ◪ 1200 ☐ 1400-2000 ☐☐ 2200-2400

Water 💧💧💧💧💧💧💧–💧💧💧💧

**Physical Activity**

Total Calories Burned

Time (10 min. increments)

| 10 | 10 | 10 |
|---|---|---|
| 10 | 10 | 10 |

Resistance Training

Upper ☐ Core ☐ Lower ☐

Week 3

## Daily Nutrition & Activity Record

Mon Tue Wed Thu Fri Sat Sun    Date:

Goal or Action for the Day:

| Food & Beverage | Amount Vol. Wt/# | Calories |
|---|---|---|
| | | |
| | | |
| | | |
| | | |
| | | |
| | | |
| | | |
| | | |
| | | |
| | | |
| | | |
| | | |
| | | |
| | | |
| | | |
| | | |
| | | |
| | | |
| | | |
| | | |
| | | |
| | | |
| | | |
| | | |
| | | |
| | | Total |

**# of Servings by Calorie Level**

1200 1400 1600 1800 2000 2200 2400

Grains

Fruits

Veggies

Dairy

Protein

Fats/Oils

Legumes 1200-1800 2000-2400

Nuts & Seeds 1200 1400-2000 2200-2400

Water

**Physical Activity**

Total Calories Burned

Time (10 min. increments)

10 10 10
10 10 10

Resistance Training

Upper Core Lower

Week 3

# Daily Nutrition & Activity Record

Mon Tue Wed Thu Fri Sat Sun Date:

Goal or Action for the Day:

| Food & Beverage | Amount Vol. Wt/# | Calories |
|---|---|---|
| | | |
| | Total | |

Week 3

**# of Servings by Calorie Level**

| | | | 1200 | | 1400 | 1600 | 1800 | 2000 | 2200 | 2400 |
|---|---|---|---|---|---|---|---|---|---|---|
| Grains | ☐ | ☐ | ☐ | +☐ | ☐ | +☐ | +☐ | +☐ | +☐ | +☐ |
| Fruits | | ☐ | ☐ | | | | +☐ | | | |
| Veggies | ☐ | ☐ | ☐ | | | +☐ | | +☐ | | +☐ |
| Dairy | ☐ | ☐ | ☐ | | | | | | | |
| Protein | ☐ ☐ | ☐ | ☐ | | | +☐ | | | | +☐ |
| Fats/Oils | | ☐ | ☐ | | | | +☐ | | | |

Legumes ◪ 1200-1800 ☐ 2000-2400

Nuts & Seeds ◪ 1200 ☐ 1400-2000 ☐☐ 2200-2400

Water ○○○○○○○○–○○○○

**Physical Activity**

Total Calories Burned

Time (10 min. increments)

| 10 | 10 | 10 |
|---|---|---|
| 10 | 10 | 10 |

Resistance Training

| Upper | Core | Lower |
|---|---|---|
| ☐ | ☐ | ☐ |

# Daily Nutrition & Activity Record

Mon Tue Wed Thu Fri Sat Sun Date:

Goal or Action for the Day:

| Food & Beverage | Amount Vol. Wt/# | Calories |
|---|---|---|
| | | |
| | | |
| | | |
| | | |
| | | |
| | | |
| | | |
| | | |
| | | |
| | | |
| | | |
| | | |
| | | |
| | | |
| | | |
| | | |
| | | |
| | | |
| | | |
| | | |
| | | |
| | | |
| | | |
| | | |
| | | |
| | | |
| | Total | |

## # of Servings by Calorie Level

| | | | | 1200 | | 1400 | 1600 | 1800 | 2000 | 2200 | 2400 |
|---|---|---|---|---|---|---|---|---|---|---|---|
| Grains | | ☐ | ☐ | ☐ | +☐ | ☐ | +☐ | +☐ | +☐ | +☐ | +☐ |
| Fruits | | | ☐ | ☐ | | | | +☐ | | | |
| Veggies | | ☐ | ☐ | ☐ | | | +☐ | | +☐ | | +☐ |
| Dairy | | ☐ | ☐ | ☐ | | | | | | | |
| Protein | ☐ | ☐ | ☐ | ☐ | | | +☐ | | | | +☐ |
| Fats/Oils | | | ☐ | ☐ | | | | +☐ | | | |

Legumes ◪ 1200-1800
☐ 2000-2400

Nuts & Seeds ◪ 1200
☐ 1400-2000
☐☐ 2200-2400

Water ◯◯◯◯◯◯◯◯–◯◯◯◯

**Physical Activity**

Total Calories Burned

Time (10 min. increments)

| 10 | 10 | 10 |
|---|---|---|
| 10 | 10 | 10 |

Resistance Training

Upper ☐ Core ☐ Lower ☐

Week 3

# Daily Nutrition & Activity Record

Mon Tue Wed Thu Fri Sat Sun Date:

Goal or Action for the Day:

| Food & Beverage | Amount Vol. Wt/# | Calories |
|---|---|---|
| | | |
| | | |
| | | |
| | | |
| | | |
| | | |
| | | |
| | | |
| | | |
| | | |
| | | |
| | | |
| | | |
| | | |
| | | |
| | | |
| | | |
| | | |
| | | |
| | | |
| | | |
| | | |
| | | |
| | | |
| | | |
| | | |
| | Total | |

## # of Servings by Calorie Level

1200 1400 1600 1800 2000 2200 2400

Grains

Fruits

Veggies

Dairy

Protein

Fats/Oils

Legumes 1200-1800 2000-2400

Nuts & Seeds 1200 1400-2000 2200-2400

Water

## Physical Activity

Total Calories Burned

Time (10 min. increments)

| 10 | 10 | 10 |
|---|---|---|
| 10 | 10 | 10 |

Resistance Training

Upper Core Lower

# Daily Nutrition & Activity Record

Mon Tue Wed Thu Fri Sat Sun Date:

Goal or Action for the Day:

| Food & Beverage | Amount Vol. Wt/#. | Calories |
|---|---|---|
| | | |
| | | |
| | | |
| | | |
| | | |
| | | |
| | | |
| | | |
| | | |
| | | |
| | | |
| | | |
| | | |
| | | |
| | | |
| | | |
| | | |
| | | |
| | | |
| | | |
| | | |
| | | |
| | | |
| | | |
| | | |
| | | |
| | Total | |

**# of Servings by Calorie Level**

1200 1400 1600 1800 2000 2200 2400

Grains
Fruits
Veggies
Dairy
Protein
Fats/Oils

Legumes 1200-1800 2000-2400

Nuts & Seeds 1200 1400-2000 2200-2400

Water

**Physical Activity**

Total Calories Burned

Time (10 min. increments)

| 10 | 10 | 10 |
|---|---|---|
| 10 | 10 | 10 |

Resistance Training

Upper Core Lower

Week 3

# Daily Nutrition & Activity Record

Mon Tue Wed Thu Fri Sat Sun Date:

Goal or Action for the Day:

| Food & Beverage | Amount Vol. Wt/# | Calories |
|---|---|---|
| | | |
| | Total | |

**# of Servings by Calorie Level**

Columns: 1200, 1400, 1600, 1800, 2000, 2200, 2400

Grains
Fruits
Veggies
Dairy
Protein
Fats/Oils

Legumes: 1200-1800; 2000-2400

Nuts & Seeds: 1200; 1400-2000; 2200-2400

Water

**Physical Activity**

Total Calories Burned

Time (10 min. increments)

| 10 | 10 | 10 |
|---|---|---|
| 10 | 10 | 10 |

Resistance Training

Upper Core Lower

## Weekly Reflection Form

| Date: | Weight: |
|---|---|

| Nutritional Summary | | | Physical Activity Summary | | |
|---|---|---|---|---|---|
| Day of Week | Calories Consumed | # Fruits & Vegs | Day of Week | Calories Burned | Time in minutes |
| Monday | | | Monday | | |
| Tuesday | | | Tuesday | | |
| Wednesday | | | Wednesday | | |
| Thursday | | | Thursday | | |
| Friday | | | Friday | | |
| Saturday | | | Saturday | | |
| Sunday | | | Sunday | | |
| Total | | | Total | | |

**Calculation for Projected Weight loss for the Week**

| Total Calories Consumed | ADL: (RMRx1.25x7) | Total Exercise Cals Burned | Calorie Difference | Calories in 1 pound fat | Projected Weight Loss |
|---|---|---|---|---|---|
| ______ - | ______ - | ______ = | ______ | ÷ 3,500 = | ______ lbs. |

**My Wellness Journal - Thoughts / Feelings / Questions:**

**Your Positive & Constructive Statement About Self:**

Week 3

# Daily Nutrition & Activity Record

Mon Tue Wed Thu Fri Sat Sun Date:

Goal or Action for the Day:

| Food & Beverage | Amount Vol. Wt/# | Calories |
|---|---|---|
| | | |
| | Total | |

## # of Servings by Calorie Level

| | | | 1200 | 1400 | 1600 | 1800 | 2000 | 2200 | 2400 |
|---|---|---|---|---|---|---|---|---|---|
| Grains | ☐ | ☐ | ☐ | +☐ | ☐ | +☐ | +☐ | +☐ | +☐ +☐ |
| Fruits | | ☐ | ☐ | | | +☐ | | | |
| Veggies | ☐ | ☐ | ☐ | | +☐ | | +☐ | | +☐ |
| Dairy | ☐ | ☐ | ☐ | | | | | | |
| Protein | ☐ ☐ | ☐ | ☐ | | +☐ | | | | +☐ |
| Fats/Oils | | ☐ | ☐ | | | +☐ | | | |

Legumes: ◪ 1200-1800; ☐ 2000-2400

Nuts & Seeds: ◪ 1200; ☐ 1400-2000; ☐☐ 2200-2400

Water ◯◯◯◯◯◯◯◯–◯◯◯◯

**Physical Activity**

Total Calories Burned

Time (10 min. increments)

| 10 | 10 | 10 |
|---|---|---|
| 10 | 10 | 10 |

Resistance Training

Upper ☐ Core ☐ Lower ☐

Week 4

# Daily Nutrition & Activity Record

Mon Tue Wed Thu Fri Sat Sun Date:

Goal or Action for the Day:

| Food & Beverage | Amount Vol. Wt/# | Calories |
|---|---|---|
| | | |
| | | |
| | | |
| | | |
| | | |
| | | |
| | | |
| | | |
| | | |
| | | |
| | | |
| | | |
| | | |
| | | |
| | | |
| | | |
| | | |
| | | |
| | | |
| | | |
| | | |
| | | |
| | | |
| | | |
| | | |
| | | |
| | Total | |

## # of Servings by Calorie Level

1200 1400 1600 1800 2000 2200 2400

Grains
Fruits
Veggies
Dairy
Protein
Fats/Oils

Legumes 1200-1800 2000-2400

Nuts & Seeds 1200 1400-2000 2200-2400

Water

**Physical Activity**

Total Calories Burned

Time (10 min. increments)

10 10 10
10 10 10

Resistance Training

Upper Core Lower

Week 4

# Daily Nutrition & Activity Record

Mon Tue Wed Thu Fri Sat Sun Date:

Goal or Action for the Day:

| Food & Beverage | Amount Vol. Wt/# | Calories |
|---|---|---|
| | | |
| | Total | |

Week 4

**# of Servings by Calorie Level**

| | | | 1200 | | 1400 | 1600 | 1800 | 2000 | 2200 | 2400 |
|---|---|---|---|---|---|---|---|---|---|---|
| Grains | ☐ | ☐ | ☐ | + ☐ | ☐ | + ☐ | + ☐ | + ☐ | + ☐ | + ☐ |
| Fruits | | ☐ | ☐ | | | | + ☐ | | | |
| Veggies | ☐ | ☐ | ☐ | | | + ☐ | | + ☐ | | + ☐ |
| Dairy | ☐ | ☐ | ☐ | | | | | | | |
| Protein | ☐ ☐ | ☐ | ☐ | | | + ☐ | | | | + ☐ |
| Fats/Oils | | ☐ | ☐ | | | | + ☐ | | | |

Legumes ◩ 1200-1800 ☐ 2000-2400

Nuts & Seeds ◩ 1200 ☐ 1400-2000 ☐☐ 2200-2400

Water 💧💧💧💧💧💧💧💧–💧💧💧💧

**Physical Activity**

Total Calories Burned

Time (10 min. increments)

| 10 | 10 | 10 |
|---|---|---|
| 10 | 10 | 10 |

Resistance Training

Upper ☐ Core ☐ Lower ☐

# Daily Nutrition & Activity Record

Mon Tue Wed Thu Fri Sat Sun Date:

Goal or Action for the Day:

| Food & Beverage | Amount Vol. Wt/# | Calories |
|---|---|---|
| | | |
| | | |
| | | |
| | | |
| | | |
| | | |
| | | |
| | | |
| | | |
| | | |
| | | |
| | | |
| | | |
| | | |
| | | |
| | | |
| | | |
| | | |
| | | |
| | | |
| | | |
| | | |
| | | |
| | | |
| | | |
| | | |
| | Total | |

## # of Servings by Calorie Level

| | | | 1200 | 1400 | 1600 | 1800 | 2000 | 2200 | 2400 |
|---|---|---|---|---|---|---|---|---|---|
| Grains | ☐ | ☐ | ☐ | +☐ | ☐ | +☐ | +☐ | +☐ | +☐ |
| Fruits | | ☐ | ☐ | | | +☐ | | | |
| Veggies | ☐ | ☐ | ☐ | | +☐ | | +☐ | | +☐ |
| Dairy | ☐ | ☐ | ☐ | | | | | | |
| Protein | ☐ ☐ | ☐ | ☐ | | +☐ | | | | +☐ |
| Fats/Oils | | ☐ | ☐ | | | +☐ | | | |

Legumes ◩ 1200-1800 ☐ 2000-2400

Nuts & Seeds ◩ 1200 ☐ 1400-2000 ☐☐ 2200-2400

Water ◯◯◯◯◯◯◯◯–◯◯◯◯

**Physical Activity**

Total Calories Burned

Time (10 min. increments)

| 10 | 10 | 10 |
|---|---|---|
| 10 | 10 | 10 |

Resistance Training

Upper ☐ Core ☐ Lower ☐

Week 4

# Daily Nutrition & Activity Record

Mon Tue Wed Thu Fri Sat Sun Date:

Goal or Action for the Day:

| Food & Beverage | Amount Vol. Wt/# | Calories |
|---|---|---|
| | | |
| | | |
| | | |
| | | |
| | | |
| | | |
| | | |
| | | |
| | | |
| | | |
| | | |
| | | |
| | | |
| | | |
| | | |
| | | |
| | | |
| | | |
| | | |
| | | |
| | | |
| | | |
| | | |
| | | |
| | | |
| | | |
| | Total | |

**# of Servings by Calorie Level**

1200 1400 1600 1800 2000 2200 2400

Grains ☐ ☐ ☐+☐ ☐+☐+☐+☐+☐+☐

Fruits ☐ ☐ +☐

Veggies ☐ ☐ ☐ +☐ +☐ +☐

Dairy ☐ ☐ ☐

Protein ☐ ☐ ☐ ☐ +☐ +☐

Fats/Oils ☐ ☐ +☐

Legumes ◪ 1200-1800 ☐ 2000-2400

Nuts & Seeds ◪ 1200 ☐ 1400-2000 ☐☐ 2200-2400

Water 💧💧💧💧💧💧💧💧–💧💧💧💧

**Physical Activity**

Total Calories Burned

Time (10 min. increments)

| 10 | 10 | 10 |
|---|---|---|
| 10 | 10 | 10 |

Resistance Training

Upper ☐ Core ☐ Lower ☐

Week 4

# Daily Nutrition & Activity Record

Mon Tue Wed Thu Fri Sat Sun Date:

Goal or Action for the Day:

| Food & Beverage | Amount Vol. Wt/# | Calories |
|---|---|---|
| | | |
| | | |
| | | |
| | | |
| | | |
| | | |
| | | |
| | | |
| | | |
| | | |
| | | |
| | | |
| | | |
| | | |
| | | |
| | | |
| | | |
| | | |
| | | |
| | | |
| | | |
| | | |
| | | |
| | | |
| | | |
| | | |
| | | |
| | Total | |

**# of Servings by Calorie Level**

| | | | | 1200 | 1400 | 1600 | 1800 | 2000 | 2200 | 2400 |
|---|---|---|---|---|---|---|---|---|---|---|
| Grains | | ☐ | ☐ | ☐ | +☐ | ☐ | +☐ | +☐ | +☐ | +☐ | +☐ |
| Fruits | | | ☐ | ☐ | | | +☐ | | | |
| Veggies | | ☐ | ☐ | ☐ | | +☐ | | +☐ | | +☐ |
| Dairy | | ☐ | ☐ | ☐ | | | | | | |
| Protein | ☐ | ☐ | ☐ | ☐ | | +☐ | | | | +☐ |
| Fats/Oils | | | ☐ | ☐ | | | +☐ | | | |

Legumes ◪ 1200-1800 ☐ 2000-2400

Nuts & Seeds ◪ 1200 ☐ 1400-2000 ☐☐ 2200-2400

Water ○○○○○○○○–○○○○

**Physical Activity**

Total Calories Burned

Time (10 min. increments)

| 10 | 10 | 10 |
|---|---|---|
| 10 | 10 | 10 |

Resistance Training

Upper Core Lower

Week 4

# Daily Nutrition & Activity Record

Mon Tue Wed Thu Fri Sat Sun Date:

Goal or Action for the Day:

| Food & Beverage | Amount Vol. Wt/# | Calories |
|---|---|---|
| | | |
| | Total | |

**# of Servings by Calorie Level**

1200 1400 1600 1800 2000 2200 2400

Grains

Fruits

Veggies

Dairy

Protein

Fats/Oils

Legumes 1200-1800 2000-2400

Nuts & Seeds 1200 1400-2000 2200-2400

Water

**Physical Activity**

Total Calories Burned

Time (10 min. increments)

10 10 10
10 10 10

Resistance Training

Upper Core Lower

Week 4

# Weekly Reflection Form

| Date: | Weight: |
|---|---|

| **Nutritional Summary** | | | **Physical Activity Summary** | | |
|---|---|---|---|---|---|
| Day of Week | Calories Consumed | # Fruits & Vegs | Day of Week | Calories Burned | Time in minutes |
| Monday | | | Monday | | |
| Tuesday | | | Tuesday | | |
| Wednesday | | | Wednesday | | |
| Thursday | | | Thursday | | |
| Friday | | | Friday | | |
| Saturday | | | Saturday | | |
| Sunday | | | Sunday | | |
| Total | | | Total | | |

**Calculation for Projected Weight loss for the Week**

| Total Calories Consumed | ADL: (RMRx1.25x7) | Total Exercise Cals Burned | Calorie Difference | Calories in 1 pound fat | Projected Weight Loss |
|---|---|---|---|---|---|
| ________ - | ________ - | ________ = | ________ | ÷ 3,500 = | ________ lbs. |

**My Wellness Journal - Thoughts / Feelings / Questions:**

**Your Positive & Constructive Statement About Self:**

Week 4

# Daily Nutrition & Activity Record

Mon Tue Wed Thu Fri Sat Sun Date:

Goal or Action for the Day:

| Food & Beverage | Amount Vol. Wt/# | Calories |
|---|---|---|
| | | |
| | | |
| | | |
| | | |
| | | |
| | | |
| | | |
| | | |
| | | |
| | | |
| | | |
| | | |
| | | |
| | | |
| | | |
| | | |
| | | |
| | | |
| | | |
| | | |
| | | |
| | | |
| | | |
| | | |
| | | |
| | | |
| | Total | |

### # of Servings by Calorie Level

1200 1400 1600 1800 2000 2200 2400

Grains

Fruits

Veggies

Dairy

Protein

Fats/Oils

Legumes 1200-1800; 2000-2400

Nuts & Seeds 1200; 1400-2000; 2200-2400

Water

### Physical Activity

Total Calories Burned

Time (10 min. increments)

| 10 | 10 | 10 |
|---|---|---|
| 10 | 10 | 10 |

Resistance Training

Upper Core Lower

Week 5

# Daily Nutrition & Activity Record

Mon Tue Wed Thu Fri Sat Sun Date:

Goal or Action for the Day:

| Food & Beverage | Amount Vol. Wt/# | Calories |
|---|---|---|
| | | |
| | Total | |

## # of Servings by Calorie Level

| | | | | 1200 | 1400 | 1600 | 1800 | 2000 | 2200 | 2400 |
|---|---|---|---|---|---|---|---|---|---|---|
| Grains | | ☐ | ☐ | ☐ | +☐ | ☐ | +☐ | +☐ | +☐ | +☐ | +☐ |
| Fruits | | | ☐ | ☐ | | | +☐ | | | |
| Veggies | | ☐ | ☐ | ☐ | | +☐ | | +☐ | | +☐ |
| Dairy | | ☐ | ☐ | ☐ | | | | | | |
| Protein | ☐ | ☐ | ☐ | ☐ | | +☐ | | | | +☐ |
| Fats/Oils | | | ☐ | ☐ | | | +☐ | | | |

Legumes ◪ 1200-1800 ☐ 2000-2400

Nuts & Seeds ◪ 1200 ☐ 1400-2000 ☐☐ 2200-2400

Water ○○○○○○○○–○○○○

**Physical Activity**

Total Calories Burned

Time (10 min. increments)

| 10 | 10 | 10 |
|---|---|---|
| 10 | 10 | 10 |

Resistance Training

Upper ☐ Core ☐ Lower ☐

Week 5

# Daily Nutrition & Activity Record

Mon Tue Wed Thu Fri Sat Sun Date:

Goal or Action for the Day:

| Food & Beverage | Amount Vol. Wt/# | Calories |
|---|---|---|
| | | |
| | | |
| | | |
| | | |
| | | |
| | | |
| | | |
| | | |
| | | |
| | | |
| | | |
| | | |
| | | |
| | | |
| | | |
| | | |
| | | |
| | | |
| | | |
| | | |
| | | |
| | | |
| | | |
| | | |
| | | |
| | | |
| | Total | |

Week 5

## # of Servings by Calorie Level

| | | | | 1200 | | 1400 | 1600 | 1800 | 2000 | 2200 | 2400 |
|---|---|---|---|---|---|---|---|---|---|---|---|
| Grains | | ☐ | ☐ | ☐ | + ☐ | ☐ | + ☐ | + ☐ | + ☐ | + ☐ | + ☐ |
| Fruits | | | ☐ | ☐ | | | | + ☐ | | | |
| Veggies | | ☐ | ☐ | ☐ | | | + ☐ | | + ☐ | | + ☐ |
| Dairy | | ☐ | ☐ | ☐ | | | | | | | |
| Protein | ☐ | ☐ | ☐ | ☐ | | | + ☐ | | | | + ☐ |
| Fats/Oils | | | ☐ | ☐ | | | | + ☐ | | | |

Legumes: ◪ 1200-1800; ☐ 2000-2400

Nuts & Seeds: ◪ 1200; ☐ 1400-2000; ☐☐ 2200-2400

Water 💧💧💧💧💧💧💧💧–💧💧💧💧

**Physical Activity**

Total Calories Burned

Time (10 min. increments)

| 10 | 10 | 10 |
|---|---|---|
| 10 | 10 | 10 |

Resistance Training

Upper ☐ Core ☐ Lower ☐

## Daily Nutrition & Activity Record

Mon Tue Wed Thu Fri Sat Sun Date:

Goal or Action for the Day:

| Food & Beverage | Amount Vol. Wt/# | Calories |
|---|---|---|
| | | |
| | | |
| | | |
| | | |
| | | |
| | | |
| | | |
| | | |
| | | |
| | | |
| | | |
| | | |
| | | |
| | | |
| | | |
| | | |
| | | |
| | | |
| | | |
| | | |
| | | |
| | | |
| | | |
| | | |
| | | |
| | | |
| | Total | |

### # of Servings by Calorie Level

| | | | 1200 | | 1400 | 1600 | 1800 | 2000 | 2200 | 2400 |
|---|---|---|---|---|---|---|---|---|---|---|
| Grains | ☐ | ☐ | ☐ | +☐ | ☐ | +☐ | +☐ | +☐ | +☐ | +☐ |
| Fruits | | ☐ | ☐ | | | | +☐ | | | |
| Veggies | ☐ | ☐ | ☐ | | | +☐ | | +☐ | | +☐ |
| Dairy | ☐ | ☐ | ☐ | | | | | | | |
| Protein | ☐ ☐ | ☐ | ☐ | | | +☐ | | | | +☐ |
| Fats/Oils | | ☐ | ☐ | | | | +☐ | | | |

Legumes ◪ 1200-1800 ☐ 2000-2400

Nuts & Seeds ◪ 1200 ☐ 1400-2000 ☐☐ 2200-2400

Water ○○○○○○○○–○○○○

**Physical Activity**

Total Calories Burned

Time (10 min. increments)

| 10 | 10 | 10 |
|---|---|---|
| 10 | 10 | 10 |

Resistance Training

Upper ☐ Core ☐ Lower ☐

Week 5

# Daily Nutrition & Activity Record

Mon Tue Wed Thu Fri Sat Sun Date:

Goal or Action for the Day:

| Food & Beverage | Amount Vol. Wt/# | Calories |
|---|---|---|
| | | |
| | Total | |

Week 5

**# of Servings by Calorie Level**

1200 1400 1600 1800 2000 2200 2400

Grains
Fruits
Veggies
Dairy
Protein
Fats/Oils

Legumes 1200-1800 2000-2400

Nuts & Seeds 1200 1400-2000 2200-2400

Water

**Physical Activity**

Total Calories Burned

Time (10 min. increments)

| 10 | 10 | 10 |
|---|---|---|
| 10 | 10 | 10 |

Resistance Training

Upper Core Lower

## Daily Nutrition & Activity Record

Mon Tue Wed Thu Fri Sat Sun Date:

Goal or Action for the Day:

| Food & Beverage | Amount Vol. Wt/# | Calories |
|---|---|---|
| | | |
| | | |
| | | |
| | | |
| | | |
| | | |
| | | |
| | | |
| | | |
| | | |
| | | |
| | | |
| | | |
| | | |
| | | |
| | | |
| | | |
| | | |
| | | |
| | | |
| | | |
| | | |
| | | |
| | | |
| | | |
| | | |
| | Total | |

### # of Servings by Calorie Level

| | | | | 1200 | 1400 | 1600 | 1800 | 2000 | 2200 | 2400 |
|---|---|---|---|---|---|---|---|---|---|---|
| Grains | | ☐ | ☐ | ☐ | +☐ | ☐ | +☐ | +☐ | +☐ | +☐ +☐ |
| Fruits | | | ☐ | ☐ | | | +☐ | | | |
| Veggies | | ☐ | ☐ | ☐ | | +☐ | | +☐ | | +☐ |
| Dairy | | ☐ | ☐ | ☐ | | | | | | |
| Protein | ☐ | ☐ | ☐ | ☐ | | +☐ | | | | +☐ |
| Fats/Oils | | | ☐ | ☐ | | | +☐ | | | |

Legumes ◩ 1200-1800 ☐ 2000-2400

Nuts & Seeds ◩ 1200 ☐ 1400-2000 ☐☐ 2200-2400

Water ◯◯◯◯◯◯◯◯–◯◯◯◯

**Physical Activity**

Total Calories Burned

Time (10 min. increments)

| 10 | 10 | 10 |
|---|---|---|
| 10 | 10 | 10 |

Resistance Training

Upper ☐ Core ☐ Lower ☐

Week 5

# Daily Nutrition & Activity Record

Mon Tue Wed Thu Fri Sat Sun Date:

Goal or Action for the Day:

| Food & Beverage | Amount Vol. Wt/# | Calories |
|---|---|---|
| | | |
| | Total | |

## # of Servings by Calorie Level

| | | | | 1200 | | 1400 | 1600 | 1800 | 2000 | 2200 | 2400 |
|---|---|---|---|---|---|---|---|---|---|---|---|
| Grains | | ☐ | ☐ | ☐ | +☐ | ☐ | +☐ | +☐ | +☐ | +☐ | +☐ |
| Fruits | | | ☐ | ☐ | | | | +☐ | | | |
| Veggies | | ☐ | ☐ | ☐ | | | +☐ | | +☐ | | +☐ |
| Dairy | | ☐ | ☐ | ☐ | | | | | | | |
| Protein | ☐ | ☐ | ☐ | ☐ | | | +☐ | | | | +☐ |
| Fats/Oils | | | ☐ | ☐ | | | | +☐ | | | |

Legumes ◪ 1200-1800 ☐ 2000-2400

Nuts & Seeds ◪ 1200 ☐ 1400-2000 ☐☐ 2200-2400

Water ○○○○○○○○–○○○○

**Physical Activity**

Total Calories Burned

Time (10 min. increments)

| 10 | 10 | 10 |
|---|---|---|
| 10 | 10 | 10 |

Resistance Training

Upper ☐ Core ☐ Lower ☐

Week 5

# Weekly Reflection Form

| Date: | Weight: |
|---|---|

| Nutritional Summary | | | Physical Activity Summary | | |
|---|---|---|---|---|---|
| Day of Week | Calories Consumed | # Fruits & Vegs | Day of Week | Calories Burned | Time in minutes |
| Monday | | | Monday | | |
| Tuesday | | | Tuesday | | |
| Wednesday | | | Wednesday | | |
| Thursday | | | Thursday | | |
| Friday | | | Friday | | |
| Saturday | | | Saturday | | |
| Sunday | | | Sunday | | |
| Total | | | Total | | |

**Calculation for Projected Weight loss for the Week**

| Total Calories Consumed | ADL: (RMRx1.25x7) | Total Exercise Cals Burned | Calorie Difference | Calories in 1 pound fat | Projected Weight Loss |
|---|---|---|---|---|---|
| ______ - | ______ - | ______ = | ______ | ÷ 3,500 = | ______ lbs. |

**My Wellness Journal - Thoughts / Feelings / Questions:**

**Your Positive & Constructive Statement About Self:**

Week 5

# Daily Nutrition & Activity Record

Mon Tue Wed Thu Fri Sat Sun Date:

Goal or Action for the Day:

| Food & Beverage | Amount Vol. Wt/# | Calories |
|---|---|---|
| | | |
| | Total | |

**# of Servings by Calorie Level**

| | | | 1200 | | 1400 | 1600 | 1800 | 2000 | 2200 | 2400 |
|---|---|---|---|---|---|---|---|---|---|---|
| Grains | ☐ | ☐ | ☐ | +☐ | ☐ | +☐ | +☐ | +☐ | +☐ | +☐ |
| Fruits | | ☐ | ☐ | | | | +☐ | | | |
| Veggies | ☐ | ☐ | ☐ | | | +☐ | | +☐ | | +☐ |
| Dairy | ☐ | ☐ | ☐ | | | | | | | |
| Protein ☐ | ☐ | ☐ | ☐ | | | +☐ | | | | +☐ |
| Fats/Oils | | ☐ | ☐ | | | | +☐ | | | |

Legumes ◪ 1200-1800 ☐ 2000-2400

Nuts & Seeds ◪ 1200 ☐ 1400-2000 ☐ ☐ 2200-2400

Water 💧💧💧💧💧💧💧💧–💧💧💧💧

**Physical Activity**

Total Calories Burned

Time (10 min. increments)

| 10 | 10 | 10 |
|---|---|---|
| 10 | 10 | 10 |

Resistance Training

Upper Core Lower

Week 6

# Daily Nutrition & Activity Record

Mon Tue Wed Thu Fri Sat Sun                Date:

Goal or Action for the Day:

| Food & Beverage | Amount | Vol. Wt/# | Calories |
|---|---|---|---|
| | | | |
| | | | |
| | | | |
| | | | |
| | | | |
| | | | |
| | | | |
| | | | |
| | | | |
| | | | |
| | | | |
| | | | |
| | | | |
| | | | |
| | | | |
| | | | |
| | | | |
| | | | |
| | | | |
| | | | |
| | | | |
| | | | |
| | | | |
| | | | |
| | | | |
| | | Total | |

**# of Servings by Calorie Level**

| | | | | 1200 | | 1400 | 1600 | 1800 | 2000 | 2200 | 2400 |
|---|---|---|---|---|---|---|---|---|---|---|---|
| Grains | | ☐ | ☐ | ☐ | +☐ | ☐ | +☐ | +☐ | +☐ | +☐ | +☐ |
| Fruits | | | ☐ | ☐ | | | | +☐ | | | |
| Veggies | | ☐ | ☐ | ☐ | | | +☐ | | +☐ | | +☐ |
| Dairy | | ☐ | ☐ | ☐ | | | | | | | |
| Protein | ☐ | ☐ | ☐ | ☐ | | | +☐ | | | | +☐ |
| Fats/Oils | | | ☐ | ☐ | | | | +☐ | | | |

Legumes ◪ 1200-1800 ☐ 2000-2400

Nuts & Seeds ◪ 1200 ☐ 1400-2000 ☐☐ 2200-2400

Water ◯◯◯◯◯◯◯◯–◯◯◯◯

**Physical Activity**

Total Calories Burned

Time (10 min. increments)

| 10 | 10 | 10 |
|---|---|---|
| 10 | 10 | 10 |

Resistance Training

Upper ☐ Core ☐ Lower ☐

Week 6

# Daily Nutrition & Activity Record

Mon Tue Wed Thu Fri Sat Sun Date:

Goal or Action for the Day:

| Food & Beverage | Amount Vol. Wt/# | Calories |
|---|---|---|
| | | |
| | | |
| | | |
| | | |
| | | |
| | | |
| | | |
| | | |
| | | |
| | | |
| | | |
| | | |
| | | |
| | | |
| | | |
| | | |
| | | |
| | | |
| | | |
| | | |
| | | |
| | | |
| | | |
| | | |
| | | |
| | | |
| | Total | |

**# of Servings by Calorie Level**

| | | | | 1200 | | 1400 | 1600 | 1800 | 2000 | 2200 | 2400 |
|---|---|---|---|---|---|---|---|---|---|---|---|
| Grains | | ☐ | ☐ | ☐ | +☐ | ☐ | +☐ | +☐ | +☐ | +☐ | +☐ |
| Fruits | | | ☐ | ☐ | | | | +☐ | | | |
| Veggies | | ☐ | ☐ | ☐ | | | +☐ | | +☐ | | +☐ |
| Dairy | | ☐ | ☐ | ☐ | | | | | | | |
| Protein | ☐ | ☐ | ☐ | ☐ | | | +☐ | | | | +☐ |
| Fats/Oils | | | ☐ | ☐ | | | | +☐ | | | |

Legumes ◩ 1200-1800
☐ 2000-2400

Nuts & Seeds ◩ 1200
☐ 1400-2000
☐☐ 2200-2400

Water 💧💧💧💧💧💧💧💧–💧💧💧💧

**Physical Activity**

Total Calories Burned

Time (10 min. increments)

| 10 | 10 | 10 |
|---|---|---|
| 10 | 10 | 10 |

Resistance Training

Upper ☐ Core ☐ Lower ☐

Week 6

# Daily Nutrition & Activity Record

Mon Tue Wed Thu Fri Sat Sun Date:

Goal or Action for the Day:

| Food & Beverage | Amount Vol. Wt/# | Calories |
|---|---|---|
| | | |
| | Total | |

**# of Servings by Calorie Level**

1200 1400 1600 1800 2000 2200 2400

Grains

Fruits

Veggies

Dairy

Protein

Fats/Oils

Legumes 1200-1800 2000-2400

Nuts & Seeds 1200 1400-2000 2200-2400

Water

**Physical Activity**

Total Calories Burned

Time (10 min. increments)

| 10 | 10 | 10 |
|---|---|---|
| 10 | 10 | 10 |

Resistance Training

Upper Core Lower

Week 6

# Daily Nutrition & Activity Record

Mon Tue Wed Thu Fri Sat Sun

Date:

Goal or Action for the Day:

| Food & Beverage | Amount Vol. Wt/# | Calories |
|---|---|---|
| | | |
| | | |
| | | |
| | | |
| | | |
| | | |
| | | |
| | | |
| | | |
| | | |
| | | |
| | | |
| | | |
| | | |
| | | |
| | | |
| | | |
| | | |
| | | |
| | | |
| | | |
| | | |
| | | |
| | | |
| | | |
| | | |
| | Total | |

## # of Servings by Calorie Level

| | | | | 1200 | | 1400 | 1600 | 1800 | 2000 | 2200 | 2400 |
|---|---|---|---|---|---|---|---|---|---|---|---|
| Grains | | ☐ | ☐ | ☐ | +☐ | ☐ | +☐ | +☐ | +☐ | +☐ | +☐ |
| Fruits | | | ☐ | ☐ | | | | +☐ | | | |
| Veggies | | ☐ | ☐ | ☐ | | | +☐ | | +☐ | | +☐ |
| Dairy | | ☐ | ☐ | ☐ | | | | | | | |
| Protein | ☐ | ☐ | ☐ | ☐ | | | +☐ | | | | +☐ |
| Fats/Oils | | | ☐ | ☐ | | | | +☐ | | | |

Legumes ◪ 1200-1800 ☐ 2000-2400

Nuts & Seeds ◪ 1200 ☐ 1400-2000 ☐☐ 2200-2400

Water 💧💧💧💧💧💧💧💧–💧💧💧💧

**Physical Activity**

Total Calories Burned

Time (10 min. increments)

| 10 | 10 | 10 |
|---|---|---|
| 10 | 10 | 10 |

Resistance Training

Upper ☐ Core ☐ Lower ☐

Week 6

# Daily Nutrition & Activity Record

Mon Tue Wed Thu Fri Sat Sun Date:

Goal or Action for the Day:

| Food & Beverage | Amount Vol. Wt/# | Calories |
|---|---|---|
| | | |
| | Total | |

## # of Servings by Calorie Level

| | | | 1200 | 1400 | 1600 | 1800 | 2000 | 2200 | 2400 |
|---|---|---|---|---|---|---|---|---|---|
| Grains | ☐ | ☐ | ☐ | +☐ | ☐ | +☐ | +☐ | +☐ | +☐ |
| Fruits | | ☐ | ☐ | | | +☐ | | | |
| Veggies | ☐ | ☐ | ☐ | | +☐ | | +☐ | | +☐ |
| Dairy | ☐ | ☐ | ☐ | | | | | | |
| Protein ☐ | ☐ | ☐ | ☐ | | +☐ | | | | +☐ |
| Fats/Oils | | ☐ | ☐ | | | +☐ | | | |

Legumes ◩ 1200-1800 ☐ 2000-2400

Nuts & Seeds ◩ 1200 ☐ 1400-2000 ☐☐ 2200-2400

Water ◯◯◯◯◯◯◯◯–◯◯◯◯

**Physical Activity**

Total Calories Burned

Time (10 min. increments)

| 10 | 10 | 10 |
|---|---|---|
| 10 | 10 | 10 |

Resistance Training

Upper ☐ Core ☐ Lower ☐

Week 6

# Daily Nutrition & Activity Record

Mon Tue Wed Thu Fri Sat Sun Date:

Goal or Action for the Day:

| Food & Beverage | Amount Vol. Wt/# | Calories |
|---|---|---|
| | | |
| | | |
| | | |
| | | |
| | | |
| | | |
| | | |
| | | |
| | | |
| | | |
| | | |
| | | |
| | | |
| | | |
| | | |
| | | |
| | | |
| | | |
| | | |
| | | |
| | | |
| | | |
| | | |
| | | |
| | | |
| | | |
| | Total | |

### # of Servings by Calorie Level

| | 1200 | 1400 | 1600 | 1800 | 2000 | 2200 | 2400 |
|---|---|---|---|---|---|---|---|
| Grains | ☐ ☐ ☐ | +☐ | ☐ | +☐ | +☐ | +☐ | +☐ |
| Fruits | ☐ ☐ | | | +☐ | | | |
| Veggies | ☐ ☐ ☐ | | +☐ | | +☐ | | +☐ |
| Dairy | ☐ ☐ ☐ | | | | | | |
| Protein | ☐ ☐ ☐ ☐ | | +☐ | | | | +☐ |
| Fats/Oils | ☐ ☐ | | | +☐ | | | |

Legumes ◪ 1200-1800 ☐ 2000-2400

Nuts & Seeds ◪ 1200 ☐ 1400-2000 ☐ ☐ 2200-2400

Water 💧💧💧💧💧💧💧💧–💧💧💧💧

**Physical Activity**

Total Calories Burned

Time (10 min. increments)

| 10 | 10 | 10 |
|---|---|---|
| 10 | 10 | 10 |

Resistance Training

Upper ☐ Core ☐ Lower ☐

Week 6

## Weekly Reflection Form

Date: | Weight:

| Nutritional Summary | | | Physical Activity Summary | | |
|---|---|---|---|---|---|
| Day of Week | Calories Consumed | # Fruits & Vegs | Day of Week | Calories Burned | Time in minutes |
| Monday | | | Monday | | |
| Tuesday | | | Tuesday | | |
| Wednesday | | | Wednesday | | |
| Thursday | | | Thursday | | |
| Friday | | | Friday | | |
| Saturday | | | Saturday | | |
| Sunday | | | Sunday | | |
| Total | | | Total | | |

**Calculation for Projected Weight loss for the Week**

| Total Calories Consumed | ADL: (RMRx1.25x7) | Total Exercise Cals Burned | Calorie Difference | Calories in 1 pound fat | Projected Weight Loss |
|---|---|---|---|---|---|
| ________ - | ________ - | ________ = | ________ | ÷ 3,500 = | ________ lbs. |

**My Wellness Journal - Thoughts / Feelings / Questions:**

**Your Positive & Constructive Statement About Self:**

Week 6

# Daily Nutrition & Activity Record

Mon Tue Wed Thu Fri Sat Sun Date:

Goal or Action for the Day:

| Food & Beverage | Amount Vol. Wt/# | Calories |
|---|---|---|
| | | |
| | | |
| | | |
| | | |
| | | |
| | | |
| | | |
| | | |
| | | |
| | | |
| | | |
| | | |
| | | |
| | | |
| | | |
| | | |
| | | |
| | | |
| | | |
| | | |
| | | |
| | | |
| | | |
| | | |
| | | |
| | | |
| | Total | |

## # of Servings by Calorie Level

1200 1400 1600 1800 2000 2200 2400

Grains

Fruits

Veggies

Dairy

Protein

Fats/Oils

Legumes 1200-1800 2000-2400

Nuts & Seeds 1200 1400-2000 2200-2400

Water

## Physical Activity

Total Calories Burned

Time (10 min. increments)

| 10 | 10 | 10 |
|---|---|---|
| 10 | 10 | 10 |

Resistance Training

Upper Core Lower

# Daily Nutrition & Activity Record

Week 7

Mon Tue Wed Thu Fri Sat Sun Date:

Goal or Action for the Day:

| Food & Beverage | Amount Vol. Wt/# | Calories |
|---|---|---|
| | | |

Total

## # of Servings by Calorie Level

1200 1400 1600 1800 2000 2200 2400

Grains
Fruits
Veggies
Dairy
Protein
Fats/Oils

Legumes 1200-1800 2000-2400

Nuts & Seeds 1200 1400-2000 2200-2400

Water

**Physical Activity**

Total Calories Burned

Time (10 min. increments)

| 10 | 10 | 10 |
|---|---|---|
| 10 | 10 | 10 |

Resistance Training

Upper Core Lower

# Daily Nutrition & Activity Record

Mon Tue Wed Thu Fri Sat Sun

Date:

Goal or Action for the Day:

| Food & Beverage | Amount Vol. Wt/# | Calories |
| --- | --- | --- |
| | | |
| | Total | |

## # of Servings by Calorie Level

| | | | 1200 | 1400 | 1600 | 1800 | 2000 | 2200 | 2400 |
| --- | --- | --- | --- | --- | --- | --- | --- | --- | --- |
| Grains | ☐ | ☐ | ☐ | +☐ | ☐ | +☐ | +☐ | +☐ | +☐ +☐ |
| Fruits | | ☐ | ☐ | | | +☐ | | | |
| Veggies | ☐ | ☐ | ☐ | | +☐ | | +☐ | | +☐ |
| Dairy | ☐ | ☐ | ☐ | | | | | | |
| Protein | ☐ ☐ | ☐ | ☐ | | +☐ | | | | +☐ |
| Fats/Oils | | ☐ | ☐ | | | +☐ | | | |

Legumes: 1200-1800; 2000-2400

Nuts & Seeds: 1200; 1400-2000; 2200-2400

Water

**Physical Activity**

Total Calories Burned

Time (10 min. increments)

| 10 | 10 | 10 |
| --- | --- | --- |
| 10 | 10 | 10 |

Resistance Training

Upper Core Lower

# Daily Nutrition & Activity Record

Week 7

Mon Tue Wed Thu Fri Sat Sun Date:

Goal or Action for the Day:

| Food & Beverage | Amount Vol. Wt/# | Calories |
|---|---|---|
| | | |
| | | |
| | | |
| | | |
| | | |
| | | |
| | | |
| | | |
| | | |
| | | |
| | | |
| | | |
| | | |
| | | |
| | | |
| | | |
| | | |
| | | |
| | | |
| | | |
| | | |
| | | |
| | | |
| | | |
| | | |
| | | |
| | Total | |

## # of Servings by Calorie Level

| | | | 1200 | | 1400 | 1600 | 1800 | 2000 | 2200 | 2400 |
|---|---|---|---|---|---|---|---|---|---|---|
| Grains | ☐ | ☐ | ☐ | +☐ | ☐ | +☐ | +☐ | +☐ | +☐ | +☐ |
| Fruits | | ☐ | ☐ | | | | +☐ | | | |
| Veggies | ☐ | ☐ | ☐ | | | +☐ | | +☐ | | +☐ |
| Dairy | ☐ | ☐ | ☐ | | | | | | | |
| Protein ☐ | ☐ | ☐ | ☐ | | | +☐ | | | | +☐ |
| Fats/Oils | | ☐ | ☐ | | | | +☐ | | | |

Legumes ◪ 1200-1800 ☐ 2000-2400

Nuts & Seeds ◪ 1200 ☐ 1400-2000 ☐☐ 2200-2400

Water 💧💧💧💧💧💧💧💧–💧💧💧💧

**Physical Activity**

Total Calories Burned

Time (10 min. increments)

| 10 | 10 | 10 |
|---|---|---|
| 10 | 10 | 10 |

Resistance Training

Upper ☐ Core ☐ Lower ☐

Week 7

# Daily Nutrition & Activity Record

Mon Tue Wed Thu Fri Sat Sun Date:

Goal or Action for the Day:

| Food & Beverage | Amount Vol. Wt/# | Calories |
|---|---|---|
| | | |
| | | |
| | | |
| | | |
| | | |
| | | |
| | | |
| | | |
| | | |
| | | |
| | | |
| | | |
| | | |
| | | |
| | | |
| | | |
| | | |
| | | |
| | | |
| | | |
| | | |
| | | |
| | | |
| | | |
| | | |
| | | |
| | Total | |

## # of Servings by Calorie Level

1200 1400 1600 1800 2000 2200 2400

Grains

Fruits

Veggies

Dairy

Protein

Fats/Oils

Legumes 1200-1800 2000-2400

Nuts & Seeds 1200 1400-2000 2200-2400

Water

**Physical Activity**

Total Calories Burned

Time (10 min. increments)

10 10 10
10 10 10

Resistance Training

Upper Core Lower

# Daily Nutrition & Activity Record

Week 7

Mon Tue Wed Thu Fri Sat Sun Date:

Goal or Action for the Day:

| Food & Beverage | Amount Vol. Wt/# | Calories |
|---|---|---|
| | | |
| | Total | |

## # of Servings by Calorie Level

| | | | 1200 | | 1400 | 1600 | 1800 | 2000 | 2200 | 2400 |
|---|---|---|---|---|---|---|---|---|---|---|
| Grains | ☐ | ☐ | ☐ | +☐ | ☐ | +☐ | +☐ | +☐ | +☐ | +☐ |
| Fruits | | ☐ | ☐ | | | | +☐ | | | |
| Veggies | ☐ | ☐ | ☐ | | | +☐ | | +☐ | | +☐ |
| Dairy | ☐ | ☐ | ☐ | | | | | | | |
| Protein ☐ | ☐ | ☐ | ☐ | | | +☐ | | | | +☐ |
| Fats/Oils | | ☐ | ☐ | | | | +☐ | | | |

Legumes ◩ 1200-1800 ☐ 2000-2400

Nuts & Seeds ◩ 1200 ☐ 1400-2000 ☐☐ 2200-2400

Water 💧💧💧💧💧💧💧💧–💧💧💧💧

**Physical Activity**

Total Calories Burned

Time (10 min. increments)

| 10 | 10 | 10 |
|---|---|---|
| 10 | 10 | 10 |

Resistance Training

Upper ☐ Core ☐ Lower ☐

Week 7

# Daily Nutrition & Activity Record

Mon Tue Wed Thu Fri Sat Sun Date:

Goal or Action for the Day:

| Food & Beverage | Amount Vol. Wt/# | Calories |
|---|---|---|
| | | |
| | | |
| | | |
| | | |
| | | |
| | | |
| | | |
| | | |
| | | |
| | | |
| | | |
| | | |
| | | |
| | | |
| | | |
| | | |
| | | |
| | | |
| | | |
| | | |
| | | |
| | | |
| | | |
| | | |
| | Total | |

## # of Servings by Calorie Level

1200 1400 1600 1800 2000 2200 2400

Grains
Fruits
Veggies
Dairy
Protein
Fats/Oils

Legumes: 1200-1800; 2000-2400

Nuts & Seeds: 1200; 1400-2000; 2200-2400

Water

**Physical Activity**

Total Calories Burned

Time (10 min. increments)

10 10 10
10 10 10

Resistance Training

Upper Core Lower

# Weekly Reflection Form

Week 7

| Date: | | | Weight: | | |
|---|---|---|---|---|---|
| **Nutritional Summary** | | | **Physical Activity Summary** | | |
| Day of Week | Calories Consumed | # Fruits & Vegs | Day of Week | Calories Burned | Time in minutes |
| Monday | | | Monday | | |
| Tuesday | | | Tuesday | | |
| Wednesday | | | Wednesday | | |
| Thursday | | | Thursday | | |
| Friday | | | Friday | | |
| Saturday | | | Saturday | | |
| Sunday | | | Sunday | | |
| Total | | | Total | | |

**Calculation for Projected Weight loss for the Week**

| Total Calories Consumed | ADL: (RMRx1.25x7) | Total Exercise Cals Burned | Calorie Difference | Calories in 1 pound fat | Projected Weight Loss |
|---|---|---|---|---|---|
| ________ - | ________ - | ________ = | ________ | ÷ 3,500 = | ________ lbs. |

**My Wellness Journal - Thoughts / Feelings / Questions:**

**Your Positive & Constructive Statement About Self:**

Week 8

# Daily Nutrition & Activity Record

Mon Tue Wed Thu Fri Sat Sun Date:

Goal or Action for the Day:

| Food & Beverage | Amount Vol. Wt/# | Calories |
|---|---|---|
| | | |
| | | |
| | | |
| | | |
| | | |
| | | |
| | | |
| | | |
| | | |
| | | |
| | | |
| | | |
| | | |
| | | |
| | | |
| | | |
| | | |
| | | |
| | | |
| | | |
| | | |
| | | |
| | | |
| | | |
| | | |
| | | |
| | | |
| | Total | |

**# of Servings by Calorie Level**

| | | | | | 1200 | | 1400 | 1600 | 1800 | 2000 | 2200 | 2400 |
|---|---|---|---|---|---|---|---|---|---|---|---|---|
| Grains | | ☐ | ☐ | ☐ | +☐ | ☐ | +☐ | +☐ | +☐ | +☐ | +☐ | |
| Fruits | | | ☐ | ☐ | | | | +☐ | | | | |
| Veggies | | ☐ | ☐ | ☐ | | | +☐ | | +☐ | | +☐ | |
| Dairy | | ☐ | ☐ | ☐ | | | | | | | | |
| Protein | ☐ | ☐ | ☐ | ☐ | | | +☐ | | | | +☐ | |
| Fats/Oils | | | ☐ | ☐ | | | | +☐ | | | | |

Legumes ◪ 1200-1800 ☐ 2000-2400

Nuts & Seeds ◪ 1200 ☐ 1400-2000 ☐☐ 2200-2400

Water 💧💧💧💧💧💧💧💧–💧💧💧💧

**Physical Activity**

Total Calories Burned

Time (10 min. increments)

| 10 | 10 | 10 |
|---|---|---|
| 10 | 10 | 10 |

Resistance Training

Upper ☐ Core ☐ Lower ☐

# Daily Nutrition & Activity Record

Mon Tue Wed Thu Fri Sat Sun Date:

Goal or Action for the Day:

| Food & Beverage | Amount Vol. Wt/# | Calories |
|---|---|---|
| | | |

Total

## # of Servings by Calorie Level

1200 1400 1600 1800 2000 2200 2400

Grains

Fruits

Veggies

Dairy

Protein

Fats/Oils

Legumes 1200-1800 2000-2400

Nuts & Seeds 1200 1400-2000 2200-2400

Water

**Physical Activity**

Total Calories Burned

Time (10 min. increments)

| 10 | 10 | 10 |
|---|---|---|
| 10 | 10 | 10 |

Resistance Training

Upper Core Lower

Week 8

Week 8

# Daily Nutrition & Activity Record

Mon Tue Wed Thu Fri Sat Sun Date:

Goal or Action for the Day:

| Food & Beverage | Amount Vol. Wt/# | Calories |
|---|---|---|
| | | |
| | | |
| | | |
| | | |
| | | |
| | | |
| | | |
| | | |
| | | |
| | | |
| | | |
| | | |
| | | |
| | | |
| | | |
| | | |
| | | |
| | | |
| | | |
| | | |
| | | |
| | | |
| | | |
| | | |
| | | |
| | | |
| | Total | |

## # of Servings by Calorie Level

| | | | 1200 | | 1400 | 1600 | 1800 | 2000 | 2200 | 2400 |
|---|---|---|---|---|---|---|---|---|---|---|
| Grains | | ☐ | ☐ | ☐ | + ☐ | ☐ | + ☐ | + ☐ | + ☐ | + ☐ |
| Fruits | | | ☐ | ☐ | | | | + ☐ | | |
| Veggies | | ☐ | ☐ | ☐ | | + ☐ | | + ☐ | | + ☐ |
| Dairy | | ☐ | ☐ | ☐ | | | | | | |
| Protein | ☐ | ☐ | ☐ | ☐ | | + ☐ | | | | + ☐ |
| Fats/Oils | | | ☐ | ☐ | | | + ☐ | | | |

Legumes ◪ 1200-1800 ☐ 2000-2400

Nuts & Seeds ◪ 1200 ☐ 1400-2000 ☐☐ 2200-2400

Water ○○○○○○○○–○○○○

**Physical Activity**

Total Calories Burned

Time (10 min. increments)

| 10 | 10 | 10 |
|---|---|---|
| 10 | 10 | 10 |

Resistance Training

Upper Core Lower

# Daily Nutrition & Activity Record

Mon Tue Wed Thu Fri Sat Sun Date:

Goal or Action for the Day:

| Food & Beverage | Amount Vol. Wt/# | Calories |
|---|---|---|
| | | |
| | Total | |

## # of Servings by Calorie Level

| | | | 1200 | 1400 | 1600 | 1800 | 2000 | 2200 | 2400 |
|---|---|---|---|---|---|---|---|---|---|
| Grains | ☐ | ☐ | ☐ | +☐ | ☐ | +☐ | +☐ | +☐ | +☐ +☐ |
| Fruits | | ☐ | ☐ | | | +☐ | | | |
| Veggies | ☐ | ☐ | ☐ | | +☐ | | +☐ | | +☐ |
| Dairy | ☐ | ☐ | ☐ | | | | | | |
| Protein | ☐ ☐ | ☐ | ☐ | | +☐ | | | | +☐ |
| Fats/Oils | | ☐ | ☐ | | | +☐ | | | |

Legumes ◪ 1200-1800 ☐ 2000-2400

Nuts & Seeds ◪ 1200 ☐ 1400-2000 ☐☐ 2200-2400

Water ◯◯◯◯◯◯◯◯–◯◯◯◯

**Physical Activity**

Total Calories Burned

Time (10 min. increments)

| 10 | 10 | 10 |
|---|---|---|
| 10 | 10 | 10 |

Resistance Training

Upper Core Lower

Week 8

Week 8

# Daily Nutrition & Activity Record

Mon Tue Wed Thu Fri Sat Sun Date:

Goal or Action for the Day:

| Food & Beverage | Amount Vol. Wt/# | Calories |
|---|---|---|
| | | |
| | | |
| | | |
| | | |
| | | |
| | | |
| | | |
| | | |
| | | |
| | | |
| | | |
| | | |
| | | |
| | | |
| | | |
| | | |
| | | |
| | | |
| | | |
| | | |
| | | |
| | | |
| | | |
| | | |
| | | |
| | | |
| | Total | |

## # of Servings by Calorie Level

1200 1400 1600 1800 2000 2200 2400

Grains

Fruits

Veggies

Dairy

Protein

Fats/Oils

Legumes 1200-1800 2000-2400

Nuts & Seeds 1200 1400-2000 2200-2400

Water

**Physical Activity**

Total Calories Burned

Time (10 min. increments)

| 10 | 10 | 10 |
|---|---|---|
| 10 | 10 | 10 |

Resistance Training

Upper Core Lower

# Daily Nutrition & Activity Record

Mon Tue Wed Thu Fri Sat Sun Date:

Goal or Action for the Day:

| Food & Beverage | Amount Vol. Wt/# | Calories |
|---|---|---|
| | | |
| | Total | |

Week 8

## # of Servings by Calorie Level

| | | | 1200 | 1400 | 1600 | 1800 | 2000 | 2200 | 2400 |
|---|---|---|---|---|---|---|---|---|---|
| Grains | ☐ | ☐ | ☐ | +☐ | ☐ | +☐ | +☐ | +☐ | +☐ +☐ |
| Fruits | | ☐ | ☐ | | | +☐ | | | |
| Veggies | ☐ | ☐ | ☐ | | +☐ | | +☐ | | +☐ |
| Dairy | ☐ | ☐ | ☐ | | | | | | |
| Protein | ☐ ☐ | ☐ | ☐ | | +☐ | | | | +☐ |
| Fats/Oils | | ☐ | ☐ | | | +☐ | | | |

Legumes ◪ 1200-1800 ☐ 2000-2400

Nuts & Seeds ◪ 1200 ☐ 1400-2000 ☐☐ 2200-2400

Water 💧💧💧💧💧💧💧💧–💧💧💧💧

**Physical Activity**

Total Calories Burned

Time (10 min. increments)

| 10 | 10 | 10 |
|---|---|---|
| 10 | 10 | 10 |

Resistance Training

Upper ☐ Core ☐ Lower ☐

Week 8

# Daily Nutrition & Activity Record

Mon Tue Wed Thu Fri Sat Sun Date:

Goal or Action for the Day:

| Food & Beverage | Amount Vol. Wt/# | Calories |
|---|---|---|
| | | |
| | Total | |

## # of Servings by Calorie Level

| | | | 1200 | | 1400 | 1600 | 1800 | 2000 | 2200 | 2400 |
|---|---|---|---|---|---|---|---|---|---|---|
| Grains | ☐ | ☐ | ☐ | +☐ | ☐ | +☐ | +☐ | +☐ | +☐ | +☐ |
| Fruits | | ☐ | ☐ | | | | +☐ | | | |
| Veggies | ☐ | ☐ | ☐ | | | +☐ | | +☐ | | +☐ |
| Dairy | ☐ | ☐ | ☐ | | | | | | | |
| Protein ☐ | ☐ | ☐ | ☐ | | | +☐ | | | | +☐ |
| Fats/Oils | | ☐ | ☐ | | | | +☐ | | | |

Legumes ◩ 1200-1800 ☐ 2000-2400

Nuts & Seeds ◩ 1200 ☐ 1400-2000 ☐☐ 2200-2400

Water 💧💧💧💧💧💧💧💧–💧💧💧💧

**Physical Activity**

Total Calories Burned

Time (10 min. increments)

| 10 | 10 | 10 |
|---|---|---|
| 10 | 10 | 10 |

Resistance Training

Upper ☐ Core ☐ Lower ☐

## Weekly Reflection Form

| Date: | | | Weight: | | |
|---|---|---|---|---|---|
| **Nutritional Summary** | | | **Physical Activity Summary** | | |
| Day of Week | Calories Consumed | # Fruits & Vegs | Day of Week | Calories Burned | Time in minutes |
| Monday | | | Monday | | |
| Tuesday | | | Tuesday | | |
| Wednesday | | | Wednesday | | |
| Thursday | | | Thursday | | |
| Friday | | | Friday | | |
| Saturday | | | Saturday | | |
| Sunday | | | Sunday | | |
| Total | | | Total | | |

**Calculation for Projected Weight loss for the Week**

| Total Calories Consumed | ADL: (RMRx1.25x7) | Total Exercise Cals Burned | Calorie Difference | Calories in 1 pound fat | Projected Weight Loss |
|---|---|---|---|---|---|
| ________ - | ________ - | ________ = | ________ | ÷ 3,500 = | ________ lbs. |

**My Wellness Journal - Thoughts / Feelings / Questions:**

**Your Positive & Constructive Statement About Self:**

Week 8

# Step 7
# Some Tools of the Trade

## Menu Plans

To help you in your preparation of eating according to your specific nutritional plan calorie level, two sample menus for each of the nutritional plan calorie levels (1200 through 2000) are provided to give you an idea of how to develop your own daily menu plans. (Found on pages 114 to 120) Blank menu plans are also provided for you to "build" additional daily menu plans for your specific calorie level customized to your unique likes and food preferences. While only a few blank forms are included, you are encouraged to build several other customized daily menu plans to both learn from the experience and provide you with a variety of selections from which to choose. Also, a form is provided for building five breakfast, 5 lunch, and 5 dinner meal plans (Found on page 121). The convenience of having these already developed meal plans with associated calorie values can prove helpful as you plan ahead for your weight loss or weight management efforts of the coming day.

## Weekly Grocery List – Page 122

## Helpful Resources – Page 139

| Sample Daily Menu Plan: 1200 Calories | |
|---|---|
| **Food Item** | **Calories** |
| **Breakfast** | |
| 1 oz oatmeal | 100 |
| 1/2 Tbl. flaxseed | 20 |
| 8oz. glass of skim milk | 86 |
| 1/2 banana | 60 |
| | |
| **Total** | **266** |
| **Morning Snack** | |
| 1 medium apple | 93 |
| 1 Tbl. peanut butter | 95 |
| | |
| **Total** | **188** |
| **Lunch** | |
| 2 slices whole wheat bread | 140 |
| 1 cup lettuce | 10 |
| 2 oz turkey | 108 |
| 1 Tbl. light mayo | 50 |
| 1 oz provalone cheese | 100 |
| | |
| **Total** | **408** |
| **Afternoon or Evening Snack** | |
| 3 stocks celery | 30 |
| 1 Tbl. Low fat Ranch dressing | 45 |
| | |
| **Total** | **75** |
| **Dinner** | |
| 1/2 cup mixed vegetables | 60 |
| 2 oz chicken breast | 80 |
| 1/2 cup cooked pinto beans | 110 |
| | |
| | |
| | |
| | |
| **Total** | **250** |
| **Total Calories for the Day** | **1187** |

| # Servings from the food groups | |
|---|---|
| Grains = 3 | Fruits = 2 |
| Vegetables = 2 1/2 | Dairy = 2 |
| Protein = 5 | Legumes = 1 |
| Nuts/Seeds = 0 | Oils = 2 |

| Sample Daily Menu Plan: 1200 Calories | |
|---|---|
| **Food Item** | **Calories** |
| **Breakfast** | |
| 1 cup skim milk | 86 |
| 1 medium apple | 93 |
| 1 oz oatmeal | 100 |
| | |
| | |
| **Total** | **279** |
| **Morning Snack** | |
| | |
| | |
| | |
| **Total** | |
| **Lunch** | |
| 10 baby carrots | 25 |
| 1 oz cheddar cheese | 114 |
| 1 oz ham | 82 |
| 1 oz lettuce | 10 |
| 2 slices whole wheat bread 140 | |
| 1 Tbl. Fat-free mayonnaise | 10 |
| **Total** | **381** |
| **Afternoon or Evening Snack** | |
| 1 Tbl. Almonds | 41 |
| 1 cup vanilla yogurt | 193 |
| | |
| **Total** | **234** |
| **Dinner** | |
| 3 oz chicken breast | 140 |
| 1/2 cup cooked black beans | 109 |
| 2 cups spinach | 14 |
| 1/2 cup strawberries | 25 |
| | |
| | |
| | |
| Total | 313 |
| **Total Calories for the Day** | **1207** |

| # Servings from the food groups | |
|---|---|
| Grains = 3 | Fruits = 2 |
| Vegetables = 2 1/2 | Dairy = 3 |
| Protein = 4 | Legumes = 1 |
| Nuts/Seeds = 1/2 | Oils = 1 |

| Sample Daily Menu Plan: 1400 Calories | | |
|---|---|---|
| **Food Item** | **Calories** | |
| **Breakfast** | | |
| 1/4 cup black beans | 54 | |
| 1 egg | 72 | |
| 5 Tbl. spoons salsa | 25 | |
| 1 small whole wheat tortilla | 80 | |
| 1 cup skim milk | 86 | |
| | **Total** | **317** |
| **Morning Snack** | | |
| 1 medium apple | 93 | |
| 1 cup light yogurt | 80 | |
| | | |
| | **Total** | **173** |
| **Lunch** | | |
| 2 slices whole wheat bread | 140 | |
| 1 Tbl. peanut butter | 95 | |
| 1 Tbl. honey | 65 | |
| 1/2 oz almonds | 82 | |
| 1 cup cucumber | 16 | |
| | | |
| | **Total** | **398** |
| **Afternoon or Evening Snack** | | |
| 3 cups popcorn | 110 | |
| 1 orange | 62 | |
| | | |
| | **Total** | **172** |
| **Dinner** | | |
| 1/2 cup green beans | 22 | |
| 2 oz top sirloin | 116 | |
| 1/2 cup brown rice | 109 | |
| 1 cup skim milk | 86 | |
| | | |
| | | |
| | | |
| | **Total** | **333** |
| **Total Calories for the Day** | | **1393** |

| # Servings from the food groups | |
|---|---|
| Grains = 5 | Fruits = 2 |
| Vegetables = 2 1/2 | Dairy = 3 |
| Protein = 4 | Legumes = 1/2 |
| Nuts/Seeds = 1 | Oils = 1 |

| Sample Daily Menu Plan: 1400 Calories | | |
|---|---|---|
| **Food Item** | **Calories** | |
| **Breakfast** | | |
| 1 egg scrambled | 72 | |
| 1 cup skim milk | 86 | |
| 1 oz cooked oatmeal | 100 | |
| 1/3 cup dried cranberries | 130 | |
| | | |
| | **Total** | **388** |
| **Morning Snack** | | |
| 1 container yougurt | 80 | |
| 1/2 cup peaches | 33 | |
| | | |
| | **Total** | **113** |
| **Lunch** | | |
| 3 oz water packed tuna | 99 | |
| 2 Tbl. fat-free mayonnaise | 20 | |
| 2 leaves of lettuce | 5 | |
| 2 slices whole wheat bread | 140 | |
| 1/2 cup carrots | 26 | |
| | | |
| | **Total** | **290** |
| **Afternoon or Evening Snack** | | |
| 1/2 oz cashews | 78 | |
| 1 stick mozzarella string cheese | 80 | |
| | | |
| | **Total** | **158** |
| **Dinner** | | |
| 1 cup whole wheat spaghetti | 221 | |
| 1/2 cup Hunts tomato sauce | 40 | |
| 1/2 cup cooked corn | 66 | |
| 1/4 cup lima beans | 54 | |
| 1 medium apple | 93 | |
| | | |
| | | |
| | **Total** | **474** |
| **Total Calories for the Day** | | **1423** |

| # Servings from the food groups | |
|---|---|
| Grains = 5 | Fruits = 2 1/2 |
| Vegetables = 3 | Dairy = 3 |
| Protein = 4 | Legumes = 1/2 |
| Nuts/Seeds = 1 | Oils = 1 |

| Sample Daily Menu Plan: 1600 Calories | | |
|---|---|---|
| **Food Item** | | **Calories** |
| **Breakfast** | | |
| 2 cups skim milk | 172 | |
| 1.5 cups Kellogs Cereal | 165 | |
| 1 banana | 105 | |
| | | |
| | | |
| | **Total** | **442** |
| **Morning Snack** | | |
| | | |
| | | |
| | | |
| | **Total** | |
| **Lunch** | | |
| 1 oz cheddar cheese | 114 | |
| 1 cup Romaine lettuce | 10 | |
| 1 tsp. mustard | 3 | |
| 2 oz sliced turkey | 60 | |
| 1 orange | 62 | |
| 2 slices whole wheat bread | 140 | |
| | **Total** | **389** |
| **Afternoon or Evening Snack** | | |
| 10 baby carrots | 52 | |
| 1/2 oz pistachios | 81 | |
| | | |
| | **Total** | **133** |
| **Dinner** | | |
| 1 cup 1% milk | 102 | |
| 1 medium baked potato | 161 | |
| 1/4 cup kidney beans | 53 | |
| 1 Tbl. Butter | 100 | |
| 2 Tbl. fat free sour cream | 26 | |
| 1/2 cup steamed broccoli | 27 | |
| 1 small whole wheat roll | 60 | |
| | **Total** | **649** |
| **Total Calories for the Day** | | **1613** |
| | | |
| **# Servings from the food groups** | | |
| Grains = 5 | Fruits = 2 | |
| Vegetables = 4 | Dairy = 3 | |
| Protein = 5 | Legumes = 1/2 | |
| Nuts/Seeds = 1 | Oils = 2 | |
| | | |

| Sample Daily Menu Plan: 1600 Calories | | |
|---|---|---|
| **Food Item** | | **Calories** |
| **Breakfast** | | |
| 1 cup cooked oatmeal | 166 | |
| 1/2 cup blueberries | 42 | |
| 1 cup 1% milk | 102 | |
| | | |
| | | |
| | **Total** | **310** |
| **Morning Snack** | | |
| 1 cup (10 baby carrots) | 52 | |
| 1 string cheese | 80 | |
| | | |
| | **Total** | **132** |
| Lunch | | |
| **1 small flour tortilla** | **92** | |
| 3 oz cooked chicken | 120 | |
| 1/4 cup red peppers, 1/4 cup tom. | 33 | |
| 1/2 cup Lettuce, 1 1/2 tsp lite Ital. | 20 | |
| 1/4 cup black beans | 54 | |
| 1/2 oz almonds | 82 | |
| | **Total** | **401** |
| **Afternoon or Evening Snack** | | |
| 1 cup strawberries | 50 | |
| 1 cup low-fat yogurt | 100 | |
| | | |
| | **Total** | **150** |
| **Dinner** | | |
| 2 oz whole wheat spaghetti | 200 | |
| 3/4 cup spaghetti sauce | 105 | |
| 1 1/2 oz ground beef | 126 | |
| 1/2 cup cooked green beans | 22 | |
| 1 dinner roll | 110 | |
| 1 Tbl. light butter | 50 | |
| | | |
| | **Total** | **613** |
| **Total Calories for the Day** | | **1606** |
| | | |
| **# Servings from the food groups** | | |
| Grains = 6 | Fruits = 3 | |
| Vegetables = 3 | Dairy = 3 | |
| Protein = 4 1/2 | Legumes = 1/2 | |
| Nuts/Seeds = 1 | Oils = 1 | |
| | | |

| Sample Daily Menu Plan: 1800 Calories | |
|---|---|
| **Food Item** | **Calories** |
| **Breakfast** | |
| 1 1/2 oz oatmeal | 150 |
| 1 medium banana | 105 |
| 1 cup skim milk | 86 |
| | |
| | |
| **Total** | **341** |
| **Morning Snack** | |
| 1 granola bar | 95 |
| 1 string cheese | 80 |
| 1 cup (10 baby carrots) | 52 |
| **Total** | **227** |
| **Lunch** | |
| 2 slices whole wheat bread | 140 |
| 4 slices turkey lunch meat | 140 |
| 2 tsp. mustard | 6 |
| 1 cup spinach | 7 |
| 1 Tbl. Light dressing | 15 |
| 1 apple | 95 |
| **Total** | **403** |
| **Afternoon or Evening Snack** | |
| 1/2 cup Mandrin oranges | 52 |
| 3 oz low-fat cottage cheese | 84 |
| 1/2 oz cashews | 78 |
| **Total** | **214** |
| **Dinner** | |
| 3 oz cooked chicken breast | 120 |
| 1 cup whole wheat penne | 280 |
| 1/2 cup marinara sauce | 109 |
| 1/2 cup peas | 59 |
| 1/2 cup cooked cabbage | 17 |
| 1 Tbl. Light butter | 50 |
| | |
| **Total** | **635** |
| **Total Calories for the Day** | **1820** |

| # Servings from the food groups | |
|---|---|
| Grains = 6 1/2 | Fruits = 3 |
| Vegetables = 4 | Dairy = 3 |
| Protein = 5 | Legumes = 0 |
| Nuts/Seeds = 1 | Oils = 1 1/2 |

| Sample Daily Menu Plan: 1800 Calories | |
|---|---|
| **Food Item** | **Calories** |
| **Breakfast** | |
| 2 small whole wheat pancakes | 184 |
| 1 banana | 105 |
| 1 cup skim milk | 86 |
| 2 Tbl. Syrup | 104 |
| | |
| **Total** | **479** |
| **Morning Snack** | |
| 6 oz yogurt | 80 |
| 1/2 cup peach | 33 |
| 3 stalks celery (8 inches) | 18 |
| **Total** | **131** |
| **Lunch** | |
| 2 slices whole wheat bread | 140 |
| 2 Tbl. Peanut butter | 190 |
| 1 Tbl. Strawberry jam | 50 |
| 1 medium apple | 95 |
| | |
| | |
| **Total** | **475** |
| **Afternoon or Evening Snack** | |
| 1 cup spinach, 1/2 cup cauliflower | 27 |
| 1/4 cup beets and tomatoes | 20 |
| 1/2 oz almonds, 1 Tbl. Light dress. | 97 |
| **Total** | **144** |
| **Dinner** | |
| 1 cup skim milk | 86 |
| 3 oz cooked chicken | 120 |
| 1/4 cup pinto beans | 55 |
| 1 cup brown rice | 218 |
| 1/2 cup mixed vegetables | 55 |
| 1 dinner roll | 110 |
| | |
| **Total** | **644** |
| **Total Calories for the Day** | **1873** |

| # Servings from the food groups | |
|---|---|
| Grains = 7 | Fruits = 3 |
| Vegetables = 4 | Dairy = 3 |
| Protein = 5 | Legumes = 1/2 |
| Nuts/Seeds = 1 | Oils = 1/2 |

| Sample Daily Menu Plan: 2000 Calories | |
|---|---|
| **Food Item** | **Calories** |
| **Breakfast** | |
| 1 1/2 oz oatmeal | 150 |
| 1/2 cup strawberries | 25 |
| 1 cup 1% milk | 102 |
| 2 slices cinnamon & raisin toast | 160 |
| | |
| **Total** | **437** |
| **Morning Snack** | |
| 3 oz low-fat cottage cheese | 84 |
| 1/2 cup mandarin oranges | 52 |
| 1/2 small bagel | 93 |
| **Total** | **229** |
| **Lunch** | |
| 1 small whole wheat tortilla | 80 |
| 1 oz shredded chicken | 65 |
| 1/2 cup black beans | 109 |
| 1/2 cup cooked corn | 67 |
| 1 1/2 oz cheddar cheese | 171 |
| 6 Tbl. mild salsa | 30 |
| **Total** | **522** |
| **Afternoon or Evening Snack** | |
| 1 string cheese | 80 |
| 2 Tbl. almonds | 82 |
| 1 medium apple | 93 |
| **Total** | **255** |
| **Dinner** | |
| 4 oz sirloin steak | 232 |
| 1/2 cup mashed potatoes | 119 |
| 1/2 cup carrots | 26 |
| 1/2 cup broccoli | 16 |
| 1 dinner roll | 110 |
| 3 cups popcorn (later snack) | 93 |
| | |
| **Total** | **596** |
| **Total Calories for the Day** | **2039** |

| # Servings from the food groups | |
|---|---|
| Grains = 8 | Fruits = 3 |
| Vegetables = 4 | Dairy = 4 |
| Protein = 5 | Legumes = 1 |
| Nuts/Seeds = 1 | Oils = 0 |

| Sample Daily Menu Plan: 2000 Calories | |
|---|---|
| **Food Item** | **Calories** |
| **Breakfast** | |
| 1 1/2 oz oatmeal | 150 |
| 1 Tbl. ground flaxseed | 40 |
| 2 eggs | 144 |
| 1 medium slice turkey bacon | 42 |
| 1 medium banana | 105 |
| **Total** | **481** |
| **Morning Snack** | |
| 1 cup plain yogurt | 160 |
| 1/2 cup raspberries | 32 |
| | |
| **Total** | |
| **Lunch** | |
| 2 slices whole wheat breat | 140 |
| 2 Tbl. peanut butter | 190 |
| 1 Tbl. honey | 65 |
| 1/2 cup grapes | 31 |
| 1 cup (10 baby carrots) | 52 |
| 2 Tbl. light dressing | 60 |
| **Total** | **538** |
| **Afternoon or Evening Snack** | |
| 1/2 oz walnuts | 93 |
| 1 string cheese | 80 |
| | |
| **Total** | **173** |
| **Dinner** | |
| 3 oz lemon peppered chicken | 138 |
| 1 medium baked potato | 129 |
| 2 Tbl. non-fat sour cream | 26 |
| 1/2 cup kidney beans | 106 |
| 1 dinner roll | 110 |
| 1 cup cooked green beans | 68 |
| | |
| **Total** | **577** |
| **Total Calories for the Day** | **1961** |

| # Servings from the food groups | |
|---|---|
| Grains = 4 | Fruits = 3 |
| Vegetables = 4 | Dairy = 2 |
| Protein = 7 | Legumes = 1 |
| Nuts/Seeds = 2 | Oils = 2 |

| Build A Daily Menu Plan of ________ Calories | |
|---|---|
| **Food Item** | **Calories** |
| **Breakfast** | |
| | |
| | |
| | |
| | |
| Total | |
| **Morning Snack** | |
| | |
| | |
| Total | |
| **Lunch** | |
| | |
| | |
| | |
| | |
| | |
| Total | |
| **Afternoon or Evening Snack** | |
| | |
| | |
| Total | |
| **Dinner** | |
| | |
| | |
| | |
| | |
| | |
| | |
| Total | |
| **Total Calories for the Day** | |
| | |
| **# Servings from the food groups** | |
| Grains = ______ | Fruits = ______ |
| Vegetables = ______ | Dairy = ______ |
| Protein = ______ | Legumes = ______ |
| Nuts/Seeds = ______ | Oils = ______ |


| Build A Daily Menu Plan of ________ Calories | |
|---|---|
| **Food Item** | **Calories** |
| **Breakfast** | |
| | |
| | |
| | |
| | |
| Total | |
| **Morning Snack** | |
| | |
| | |
| Total | |
| **Lunch** | |
| | |
| | |
| | |
| | |
| | |
| Total | |
| **Afternoon or Evening Snack** | |
| | |
| | |
| Total | |
| **Dinner** | |
| | |
| | |
| | |
| | |
| | |
| | |
| Total | |
| **Total Calories for the Day** | |
| | |
| **# Servings from the food groups** | |
| Grains = ______ | Fruits = ______ |
| Vegetables = ______ | Dairy = ______ |
| Protein = ______ | Legumes = ______ |
| Nuts/Seeds = ______ | Oils = ______ |

| Build A Daily Menu Plan of ________ Calories | |
|---|---|
| Food Item | Calories |
| **Breakfast** | |
| | |
| | |
| | |
| | |
| | |
| Total | |
| **Morning Snack** | |
| | |
| | |
| | |
| Total | |
| **Lunch** | |
| | |
| | |
| | |
| | |
| | |
| | |
| Total | |
| **Afternoon or Evening Snack** | |
| | |
| | |
| | |
| Total | |
| **Dinner** | |
| | |
| | |
| | |
| | |
| | |
| | |
| | |
| Total | |
| **Total Calories for the Day** | |
| | |
| **# Servings from the food groups** | |
| Grains = ______ | Fruits = ______ |
| Vegetables = ______ | Dairy = ______ |
| Protein = ______ | Legumes = ______ |
| Nuts/Seeds = ______ | Oils = ______ |
| | |


| Build A Daily Menu Plan of ________ Calories | |
|---|---|
| Food Item | Calories |
| **Breakfast** | |
| | |
| | |
| | |
| | |
| | |
| Total | |
| **Morning Snack** | |
| | |
| | |
| | |
| Total | |
| **Lunch** | |
| | |
| | |
| | |
| | |
| | |
| | |
| Total | |
| **Afternoon or Evening Snack** | |
| | |
| | |
| | |
| Total | |
| **Dinner** | |
| | |
| | |
| | |
| | |
| | |
| | |
| | |
| Total | |
| **Total Calories for the Day** | |
| | |
| **# Servings from the food groups** | |
| Grains = ______ | Fruits = ______ |
| Vegetables = ______ | Dairy = ______ |
| Protein = ______ | Legumes = ______ |
| Nuts/Seeds = ______ | Oils = ______ |
| | |

| Breakfast Meal Plans | Cal. |
|---|---|
| 2 eggs | 144 |
| 6 Tbl. salsa | 30 |
| 1 oz cooked ham | 82 |
| 1 sl whole wheat toast | 140 |
| 1 cup skim milk | 86 |
| | |
| **Total** | **482** |
| | |
| | |
| | |
| | |
| | |
| | |
| **Total** | |
| | |
| | |
| | |
| | |
| | |
| | |
| **Total** | |
| | |
| | |
| | |
| | |
| | |
| | |
| **Total** | |
| | |
| | |
| | |
| | |
| | |
| | |
| **Total** | |
| | |
| | |
| | |
| | |
| | |
| | |
| **Total** | |

| Lunch Meal Plans | Cal. |
|---|---|
| 2 slices whole wheat bread | 140 |
| 3 oz sliced turkey | 162 |
| 2 Tbl. light salad dressing | 60 |
| 1/2 cup lettuce | 5 |
| 1 medium apple | 93 |
| | |
| **Total** | **460** |
| | |
| | |
| | |
| | |
| | |
| | |
| **Total** | |
| | |
| | |
| | |
| | |
| | |
| | |
| **Total** | |
| | |
| | |
| | |
| | |
| | |
| | |
| **Total** | |
| | |
| | |
| | |
| | |
| | |
| | |
| **Total** | |
| | |
| | |
| | |
| | |
| | |
| | |
| **Total** | |

| Dinner Meal Plans | Cal. |
|---|---|
| 3 oz grilled chicken | 120 |
| 1 cup cooked green beans | 44 |
| 2 Tbl. BBQ sauce | 70 |
| 2 oz sour dough bread | 156 |
| 2 Tbl. olive oil with garlic | 145 |
| 1/2 cup black beans | 109 |
| **Total** | **644** |
| | |
| | |
| | |
| | |
| | |
| | |
| **Total** | |
| | |
| | |
| | |
| | |
| | |
| | |
| **Total** | |
| | |
| | |
| | |
| | |
| | |
| | |
| **Total** | |
| | |
| | |
| | |
| | |
| | |
| | |
| **Total** | |
| | |
| | |
| | |
| | |
| | |
| | |
| **Total** | |

## Weekly Grocery List

Because being prepared is such an important part of a successful weight management program, a Weekly Grocery List is provided to assist you in planning the foods that you will need to purchase according to the meals you have planned or will plan to eat that week.

Note: Before you plan your meals for the week and develop your grocery list, a quick glance at the various food categories and their respective calorie amounts can be very helpful in selecting those items of lower calorie amounts.

# Weekly Grocery List

## Vegetables

- Asparagus
- Beets
- Broccoli
- Cabbage
- Carrots
- Cauliflower
- Celery
- Corn
- Cucumbers
- Lettuce/Greens
- Mushrooms
- Onions
- Peas
- Peppers
- Potatoes
- Radishes
- Spinach
- Squash
- Sweet Potatoes
- Zucchini

## Grains

- Bagels
- Barley
- Cold Cereal
- Creamed Wheat
- Dinner Rolls
- English Muffins
- French Bread
- Hamburger Buns
- Hot Dog Buns
- Macaroni Noodles
- Oatmeal
- Pancake Mix
- Pasta Noodles
- Pita Bread
- Rice (Brown)
- Rice (White)
- Spaghetti Noodles
- Tortillas
- Whole Wheat Bread Fruits

## Fruits

- Apples
- Avocado
- Bananas
- Blackberries
- Blueberries
- Cantaloupe
- Cherries
- Cranberries
- Grapefruit
- Grapes
- Honeydew
- Kiwi
- Lemons
- Limes
- Mango
- Melon
- Nectarines
- Olives
- Oranges
- Peaches
- Pears
- Pineapple
- Plums
- Raspberries
- Stawberries
- Tomatoes
- Watermelon

## Nuts & Seeds

- Almonds
- Brazil Nuts
- Cashews
- Flaxseed
- Hazelnuts
- Macadamia
- Peanuts
- Pecans
- Pine Nuts
- Pistachios
- Pumpkin Seeds
- Sesame Seeds
- Sunflower Seeds
- Walnuts

## Protein

### Seafood

- Catfish
- Clams
- Cod
- Crab
- Halibut
- Lobster
- Mussels
- Oysters
- Salmon
- Snapper
- Shrimp
- Tilapia
- Tuna

## Meat

- Bacon/ Sausage
- Beef
- Chicken
- Eggs
- Ham/Pork
- Hot Dogs
- Lunch Meat
- Steak
- Turkey

## Legumes

- Black Beans
- Black-eyed Peas
- Garbanzo Beans
- Great Northern Beans
- Kidney Beans
- Lentils
- Lima Beans
- Pinto Beans
- Red Beans
- Small White Beans
- Soybeans
- Split Peas

## Weekly Grocery List

### Dairy
- ☐ Butter/Margarine
- ☐ Cream Cheese
- ☐ Milk
- ☐ Sour Cream
- ☐ Whipped Cream
- ☐ Yogurt

### Cheese
- ☐ Bleu Cheese
- ☐ Cheddar
- ☐ Cottage Cheese
- ☐ Cream Cheese
- ☐ Feta
- ☐ Goat Cheese
- ☐ Mozzarella
- ☐ Muenster
- ☐ Parmesan
- ☐ Provolone
- ☐ Ricotta
- ☐ Swiss

### Baking/ Dry
- ☐ Baking Powder
- ☐ Baking Soda
- ☐ Bread Crumbs
- ☐ Cornmeal
- ☐ Cornstarch
- ☐ Flour
- ☐ Sugar (Brown)
- ☐ Sugar (Powder)
- ☐ Sugar (White)
- ☐ Vanilla
- ☐ Yeast

### Weight loss Helps
- ☐ Gum
- ☐ Hard Candies/Mints
- ☐ Waterbottle
- ☐ Zero Calorie Drinks

### Healthy Snacks
- ☐ Dried Fruit
- ☐ Graham Crackers
- ☐ Granola Bars
- ☐ Popcorn
- ☐ Pretzels

### Sauces/Oils
- ☐ Canola Oil
- ☐ Hot Sauce
- ☐ Olive Oil
- ☐ Soy Sauce
- ☐ Spaghetti Sauce
- ☐ Syrup
- ☐ Vegetable Oil
- ☐ Vinegar

### Canned Foods
- ☐ Applesauce
- ☐ Beans
- ☐ Broth
- ☐ Chili
- ☐ Fruits
- ☐ Soup
- ☐ Tomato Sauce

_Notes:_

### Spices & Herbs
- ☐ Basil
- ☐ Black Pepper
- ☐ Cilantro
- ☐ Cinnamon
- ☐ Garlic
- ☐ Ginger
- ☐ Mint
- ☐ Oregano
- ☐ Paprika
- ☐ Parsley
- ☐ Red Pepper
- ☐ Salt

### Condiments
- ☐ BBQ Sauce
- ☐ Croutons
- ☐ Honey
- ☐ Jam/Jelly
- ☐ Ketchup
- ☐ Mayonnaise
- ☐ Mustard
- ☐ Peanut Butter
- ☐ Pickles
- ☐ Salad Dressing
- ☐ Salsa

## Weekly Grocery List

### Vegetables
- Asparagus
- Beets
- Broccoli
- Cabbage
- Carrots
- Cauliflower
- Celery
- Corn
- Cucumbers
- Lettuce/Greens
- Mushrooms
- Onions
- Peas
- Peppers
- Potatoes
- Radishes
- Spinach
- Squash
- Sweet Potatoes
- Zucchini

### Grains
- Bagels
- Barley
- Cold Cereal
- Creamed Wheat
- Dinner Rolls
- English Muffins
- French Bread
- Hamburger Buns
- Hot Dog Buns
- Macaroni Noodles
- Oatmeal
- Pancake Mix
- Pasta Noodles
- Pita Bread
- Rice (Brown)
- Rice (White)
- Spaghetti Noodles
- Tortillas
- Whole Wheat Bread Fruits

### Fruits
- Apples
- Avocado
- Bananas
- Blackberries
- Blueberries
- Cantaloupe
- Cherries
- Cranberries
- Grapefruit
- Grapes
- Honeydew
- Kiwi
- Lemons
- Limes
- Mango
- Melon
- Nectarines
- Olives
- Oranges
- Peaches
- Pears
- Pineapple
- Plums
- Raspberries
- Stawberries
- Tomatoes
- Watermelon

### Nuts & Seeds
- Almonds
- Brazil Nuts
- Cashews
- Flaxseed
- Hazelnuts
- Macadamia
- Peanuts
- Pecans
- Pine Nuts
- Pistachios
- Pumpkin Seeds
- Sesame Seeds
- Sunflower Seeds
- Walnuts

### Protein

#### Seafood
- Catfish
- Clams
- Cod
- Crab
- Halibut
- Lobster
- Mussels
- Oysters
- Salmon
- Snapper
- Shrimp
- Tilapia
- Tuna

#### Meat
- Bacon/ Sausage
- Beef
- Chicken
- Eggs
- Ham/Pork
- Hot Dogs
- Lunch Meat
- Steak
- Turkey

#### Legumes
- Black Beans
- Black-eyed Peas
- Garbanzo Beans
- Great Northern Beans
- Kidney Beans
- Lentils
- Lima Beans
- Pinto Beans
- Red Beans
- Small White Beans
- Soybeans
- Split Peas

# Weekly Grocery List

## Dairy
- ☐ Butter/Margarine
- ☐ Cream Cheese
- ☐ Milk
- ☐ Sour Cream
- ☐ Whipped Cream
- ☐ Yogurt

## Cheese
- ☐ Bleu Cheese
- ☐ Cheddar
- ☐ Cottage Cheese
- ☐ Cream Cheese
- ☐ Feta
- ☐ Goat Cheese
- ☐ Mozzarella
- ☐ Muenster
- ☐ Parmesan
- ☐ Provolone
- ☐ Ricotta
- ☐ Swiss

## Baking/ Dry
- ☐ Baking Powder
- ☐ Baking Soda
- ☐ Bread Crumbs
- ☐ Cornmeal
- ☐ Cornstarch
- ☐ Flour
- ☐ Sugar (Brown)
- ☐ Sugar (Powder)
- ☐ Sugar (White)
- ☐ Vanilla
- ☐ Yeast

## Weight loss Helps
- ☐ Gum
- ☐ Hard Candies/Mints
- ☐ Waterbottle
- ☐ Zero Calorie Drinks

## Healthy Snacks
- ☐ Dried Fruit
- ☐ Graham Crackers
- ☐ Granola Bars
- ☐ Popcorn
- ☐ Pretzels

## Sauces/Oils
- ☐ Canola Oil
- ☐ Hot Sauce
- ☐ Olive Oil
- ☐ Soy Sauce
- ☐ Spaghetti Sauce
- ☐ Syrup
- ☐ Vegetable Oil
- ☐ Vinegar

## Canned Foods
- ☐ Applesauce
- ☐ Beans
- ☐ Broth
- ☐ Chili
- ☐ Fruits
- ☐ Soup
- ☐ Tomato Sauce

*Notes:*

## Spices & Herbs
- ☐ Basil
- ☐ Black Pepper
- ☐ Cilantro
- ☐ Cinnamon
- ☐ Garlic
- ☐ Ginger
- ☐ Mint
- ☐ Oregano
- ☐ Paprika
- ☐ Parsley
- ☐ Red Pepper
- ☐ Salt

## Condiments
- ☐ BBQ Sauce
- ☐ Croutons
- ☐ Honey
- ☐ Jam/Jelly
- ☐ Ketchup
- ☐ Mayonnaise
- ☐ Mustard
- ☐ Peanut Butter
- ☐ Pickles
- ☐ Salad Dressing
- ☐ Salsa

# Weekly Grocery List

## Vegetables

- Asparagus
- Beets
- Broccoli
- Cabbage
- Carrots
- Cauliflower
- Celery
- Corn
- Cucumbers
- Lettuce/Greens
- Mushrooms
- Onions
- Peas
- Peppers
- Potatoes
- Radishes
- Spinach
- Squash
- Sweet Potatoes
- Zucchini

## Grains

- Bagels
- Barley
- Cold Cereal
- Creamed Wheat
- Dinner Rolls
- English Muffins
- French Bread
- Hamburger Buns
- Hot Dog Buns
- Macaroni Noodles
- Oatmeal
- Pancake Mix
- Pasta Noodles
- Pita Bread
- Rice (Brown)
- Rice (White)
- Spaghetti Noodles
- Tortillas
- Whole Wheat Bread Fruits

## Fruits

- Apples
- Avocado
- Bananas
- Blackberries
- Blueberries
- Cantaloupe
- Cherries
- Cranberries
- Grapefruit
- Grapes
- Honeydew
- Kiwi
- Lemons
- Limes
- Mango
- Melon
- Nectarines
- Olives
- Oranges
- Peaches
- Pears
- Pineapple
- Plums
- Raspberries
- Stawberries
- Tomatoes
- Watermelon

## Nuts & Seeds

- Almonds
- Brazil Nuts
- Cashews
- Flaxseed
- Hazelnuts
- Macadamia
- Peanuts
- Pecans
- Pine Nuts
- Pistachios
- Pumpkin Seeds
- Sesame Seeds
- Sunflower Seeds
- Walnuts

## Protein

### Seafood

- Catfish
- Clams
- Cod
- Crab
- Halibut
- Lobster
- Mussels
- Oysters
- Salmon
- Snapper
- Shrimp
- Tilapia
- Tuna

### Meat

- Bacon/ Sausage
- Beef
- Chicken
- Eggs
- Ham/Pork
- Hot Dogs
- Lunch Meat
- Steak
- Turkey

## Legumes

- Black Beans
- Black-eyed Peas
- Garbanzo Beans
- Great Northern Beans
- Kidney Beans
- Lentils
- Lima Beans
- Pinto Beans
- Red Beans
- Small White Beans
- Soybeans
- Split Peas

## Weekly Grocery List

### Dairy
- ☐ Butter/Margarine
- ☐ Cream Cheese
- ☐ Milk
- ☐ Sour Cream
- ☐ Whipped Cream
- ☐ Yogurt

### Cheese
- ☐ Bleu Cheese
- ☐ Cheddar
- ☐ Cottage Cheese
- ☐ Cream Cheese
- ☐ Feta
- ☐ Goat Cheese
- ☐ Mozzarella
- ☐ Muenster
- ☐ Parmesan
- ☐ Provolone
- ☐ Ricotta
- ☐ Swiss

### Baking/ Dry
- ☐ Baking Powder
- ☐ Baking Soda
- ☐ Bread Crumbs
- ☐ Cornmeal
- ☐ Cornstarch
- ☐ Flour
- ☐ Sugar (Brown)
- ☐ Sugar (Powder)
- ☐ Sugar (White)
- ☐ Vanilla
- ☐ Yeast

### Weight loss Helps
- ☐ Gum
- ☐ Hard Candies/Mints
- ☐ Waterbottle
- ☐ Zero Calorie Drinks

### Healthy Snacks
- ☐ Dried Fruit
- ☐ Graham Crackers
- ☐ Granola Bars
- ☐ Popcorn
- ☐ Pretzels

### Sauces/Oils
- ☐ Canola Oil
- ☐ Hot Sauce
- ☐ Olive Oil
- ☐ Soy Sauce
- ☐ Spaghetti Sauce
- ☐ Syrup
- ☐ Vegetable Oil
- ☐ Vinegar

### Canned Foods
- ☐ Applesauce
- ☐ Beans
- ☐ Broth
- ☐ Chili
- ☐ Fruits
- ☐ Soup
- ☐ Tomato Sauce

*Notes:*

### Spices & Herbs
- ☐ Basil
- ☐ Black Pepper
- ☐ Cilantro
- ☐ Cinnamon
- ☐ Garlic
- ☐ Ginger
- ☐ Mint
- ☐ Oregano
- ☐ Paprika
- ☐ Parsley
- ☐ Red Pepper
- ☐ Salt

### Condiments
- ☐ BBQ Sauce
- ☐ Croutons
- ☐ Honey
- ☐ Jam/Jelly
- ☐ Ketchup
- ☐ Mayonnaise
- ☐ Mustard
- ☐ Peanut Butter
- ☐ Pickles
- ☐ Salad Dressing
- ☐ Salsa

# Weekly Grocery List

## Vegetables

- ☐ Asparagus
- ☐ Beets
- ☐ Broccoli
- ☐ Cabbage
- ☐ Carrots
- ☐ Cauliflower
- ☐ Celery
- ☐ Corn
- ☐ Cucumbers
- ☐ Lettuce/Greens
- ☐ Mushrooms
- ☐ Onions
- ☐ Peas
- ☐ Peppers
- ☐ Potatoes
- ☐ Radishes
- ☐ Spinach
- ☐ Squash
- ☐ Sweet Potatoes
- ☐ Zucchini

## Grains

- ☐ Bagels
- ☐ Barley
- ☐ Cold Cereal
- ☐ Creamed Wheat
- ☐ Dinner Rolls
- ☐ English Muffins
- ☐ French Bread
- ☐ Hamburger Buns
- ☐ Hot Dog Buns
- ☐ Macaroni Noodles
- ☐ Oatmeal
- ☐ Pancake Mix
- ☐ Pasta Noodles
- ☐ Pita Bread
- ☐ Rice (Brown)
- ☐ Rice (White)
- ☐ Spaghetti Noodles
- ☐ Tortillas
- ☐ Whole Wheat Bread Fruits

## Fruits

- ☐ Apples
- ☐ Avocado
- ☐ Bananas
- ☐ Blackberries
- ☐ Blueberries
- ☐ Cantaloupe
- ☐ Cherries
- ☐ Cranberries
- ☐ Grapefruit
- ☐ Grapes
- ☐ Honeydew
- ☐ Kiwi
- ☐ Lemons
- ☐ Limes
- ☐ Mango
- ☐ Melon
- ☐ Nectarines
- ☐ Olives
- ☐ Oranges
- ☐ Peaches
- ☐ Pears
- ☐ Pineapple
- ☐ Plums
- ☐ Raspberries
- ☐ Stawberries
- ☐ Tomatoes
- ☐ Watermelon

## Nuts & Seeds

- ☐ Almonds
- ☐ Brazil Nuts
- ☐ Cashews
- ☐ Flaxseed
- ☐ Hazelnuts
- ☐ Macadamia
- ☐ Peanuts
- ☐ Pecans
- ☐ Pine Nuts
- ☐ Pistachios
- ☐ Pumpkin Seeds
- ☐ Sesame Seeds
- ☐ Sunflower Seeds
- ☐ Walnuts

## Protein

### Seafood

- ☐ Catfish
- ☐ Clams
- ☐ Cod
- ☐ Crab
- ☐ Halibut
- ☐ Lobster
- ☐ Mussels
- ☐ Oysters
- ☐ Salmon
- ☐ Snapper
- ☐ Shrimp
- ☐ Tilapia
- ☐ Tuna

## Meat

- ☐ Bacon/ Sausage
- ☐ Beef
- ☐ Chicken
- ☐ Eggs
- ☐ Ham/Pork
- ☐ Hot Dogs
- ☐ Lunch Meat
- ☐ Steak
- ☐ Turkey

## Legumes

- ☐ Black Beans
- ☐ Black-eyed Peas
- ☐ Garbanzo Beans
- ☐ Great Northern Beans
- ☐ Kidney Beans
- ☐ Lentils
- ☐ Lima Beans
- ☐ Pinto Beans
- ☐ Red Beans
- ☐ Small White Beans
- ☐ Soybeans
- ☐ Split Peas

# Weekly Grocery List

## Dairy
- ☐ Butter/Margarine
- ☐ Cream Cheese
- ☐ Milk
- ☐ Sour Cream
- ☐ Whipped Cream
- ☐ Yogurt

## Cheese
- ☐ Bleu Cheese
- ☐ Cheddar
- ☐ Cottage Cheese
- ☐ Cream Cheese
- ☐ Feta
- ☐ Goat Cheese
- ☐ Mozzarella
- ☐ Muenster
- ☐ Parmesan
- ☐ Provolone
- ☐ Ricotta
- ☐ Swiss

## Baking/ Dry
- ☐ Baking Powder
- ☐ Baking Soda
- ☐ Bread Crumbs
- ☐ Cornmeal
- ☐ Cornstarch
- ☐ Flour
- ☐ Sugar (Brown)
- ☐ Sugar (Powder)
- ☐ Sugar (White)
- ☐ Vanilla
- ☐ Yeast

## Weight loss Helps
- ☐ Gum
- ☐ Hard Candies/Mints
- ☐ Waterbottle
- ☐ Zero Calorie Drinks

## Healthy Snacks
- ☐ Dried Fruit
- ☐ Graham Crackers
- ☐ Granola Bars
- ☐ Popcorn
- ☐ Pretzels

## Sauces/Oils
- ☐ Canola Oil
- ☐ Hot Sauce
- ☐ Olive Oil
- ☐ Soy Sauce
- ☐ Spaghetti Sauce
- ☐ Syrup
- ☐ Vegetable Oil
- ☐ Vinegar

## Canned Foods
- ☐ Applesauce
- ☐ Beans
- ☐ Broth
- ☐ Chili
- ☐ Fruits
- ☐ Soup
- ☐ Tomato Sauce

*Notes:*

## Spices & Herbs
- ☐ Basil
- ☐ Black Pepper
- ☐ Cilantro
- ☐ Cinnamon
- ☐ Garlic
- ☐ Ginger
- ☐ Mint
- ☐ Oregano
- ☐ Paprika
- ☐ Parsley
- ☐ Red Pepper
- ☐ Salt

## Condiments
- ☐ BBQ Sauce
- ☐ Croutons
- ☐ Honey
- ☐ Jam/Jelly
- ☐ Ketchup
- ☐ Mayonnaise
- ☐ Mustard
- ☐ Peanut Butter
- ☐ Pickles
- ☐ Salad Dressing
- ☐ Salsa

# Weekly Grocery List

## Vegetables

- ☐ Asparagus
- ☐ Beets
- ☐ Broccoli
- ☐ Cabbage
- ☐ Carrots
- ☐ Cauliflower
- ☐ Celery
- ☐ Corn
- ☐ Cucumbers
- ☐ Lettuce/Greens
- ☐ Mushrooms
- ☐ Onions
- ☐ Peas
- ☐ Peppers
- ☐ Potatoes
- ☐ Radishes
- ☐ Spinach
- ☐ Squash
- ☐ Sweet Potatoes
- ☐ Zucchini

## Grains

- ☐ Bagels
- ☐ Barley
- ☐ Cold Cereal
- ☐ Creamed Wheat
- ☐ Dinner Rolls
- ☐ English Muffins
- ☐ French Bread
- ☐ Hamburger Buns
- ☐ Hot Dog Buns
- ☐ Macaroni Noodles
- ☐ Oatmeal
- ☐ Pancake Mix
- ☐ Pasta Noodles
- ☐ Pita Bread
- ☐ Rice (Brown)
- ☐ Rice (White)
- ☐ Spaghetti Noodles
- ☐ Tortillas
- ☐ Whole Wheat Bread Fruits

## Fruits

- ☐ Apples
- ☐ Avocado
- ☐ Bananas
- ☐ Blackberries
- ☐ Blueberries
- ☐ Cantaloupe
- ☐ Cherries
- ☐ Cranberries
- ☐ Grapefruit
- ☐ Grapes
- ☐ Honeydew
- ☐ Kiwi
- ☐ Lemons
- ☐ Limes
- ☐ Mango
- ☐ Melon
- ☐ Nectarines
- ☐ Olives
- ☐ Oranges
- ☐ Peaches
- ☐ Pears
- ☐ Pineapple
- ☐ Plums
- ☐ Raspberries
- ☐ Stawberries
- ☐ Tomatoes
- ☐ Watermelon

## Nuts & Seeds

- ☐ Almonds
- ☐ Brazil Nuts
- ☐ Cashews
- ☐ Flaxseed
- ☐ Hazelnuts
- ☐ Macadamia
- ☐ Peanuts
- ☐ Pecans
- ☐ Pine Nuts
- ☐ Pistachios
- ☐ Pumpkin Seeds
- ☐ Sesame Seeds
- ☐ Sunflower Seeds
- ☐ Walnuts

## Protein

### Seafood

- ☐ Catfish
- ☐ Clams
- ☐ Cod
- ☐ Crab
- ☐ Halibut
- ☐ Lobster
- ☐ Mussels
- ☐ Oysters
- ☐ Salmon
- ☐ Snapper
- ☐ Shrimp
- ☐ Tilapia
- ☐ Tuna

### Meat

- ☐ Bacon/ Sausage
- ☐ Beef
- ☐ Chicken
- ☐ Eggs
- ☐ Ham/Pork
- ☐ Hot Dogs
- ☐ Lunch Meat
- ☐ Steak
- ☐ Turkey

### Legumes

- ☐ Black Beans
- ☐ Black-eyed Peas
- ☐ Garbanzo Beans
- ☐ Great Northern Beans
- ☐ Kidney Beans
- ☐ Lentils
- ☐ Lima Beans
- ☐ Pinto Beans
- ☐ Red Beans
- ☐ Small White Beans
- ☐ Soybeans
- ☐ Split Peas

# Weekly Grocery List

## Dairy
- ☐ Butter/Margarine
- ☐ Cream Cheese
- ☐ Milk
- ☐ Sour Cream
- ☐ Whipped Cream
- ☐ Yogurt

## Cheese
- ☐ Bleu Cheese
- ☐ Cheddar
- ☐ Cottage Cheese
- ☐ Cream Cheese
- ☐ Feta
- ☐ Goat Cheese
- ☐ Mozzarella
- ☐ Muenster
- ☐ Parmesan
- ☐ Provolone
- ☐ Ricotta
- ☐ Swiss

## Baking/ Dry
- ☐ Baking Powder
- ☐ Baking Soda
- ☐ Bread Crumbs
- ☐ Cornmeal
- ☐ Cornstarch
- ☐ Flour
- ☐ Sugar (Brown)
- ☐ Sugar (Powder)
- ☐ Sugar (White)
- ☐ Vanilla
- ☐ Yeast

## Weight loss Helps
- ☐ Gum
- ☐ Hard Candies/Mints
- ☐ Waterbottle
- ☐ Zero Calorie Drinks

## Healthy Snacks
- ☐ Dried Fruit
- ☐ Graham Crackers
- ☐ Granola Bars
- ☐ Popcorn
- ☐ Pretzels

## Sauces/Oils
- ☐ Canola Oil
- ☐ Hot Sauce
- ☐ Olive Oil
- ☐ Soy Sauce
- ☐ Spaghetti Sauce
- ☐ Syrup
- ☐ Vegetable Oil
- ☐ Vinegar

## Canned Foods
- ☐ Applesauce
- ☐ Beans
- ☐ Broth
- ☐ Chili
- ☐ Fruits
- ☐ Soup
- ☐ Tomato Sauce

*Notes:*

## Spices & Herbs
- ☐ Basil
- ☐ Black Pepper
- ☐ Cilantro
- ☐ Cinnamon
- ☐ Garlic
- ☐ Ginger
- ☐ Mint
- ☐ Oregano
- ☐ Paprika
- ☐ Parsley
- ☐ Red Pepper
- ☐ Salt

## Condiments
- ☐ BBQ Sauce
- ☐ Croutons
- ☐ Honey
- ☐ Jam/Jelly
- ☐ Ketchup
- ☐ Mayonnaise
- ☐ Mustard
- ☐ Peanut Butter
- ☐ Pickles
- ☐ Salad Dressing
- ☐ Salsa

# Weekly Grocery List

## Vegetables

- Asparagus
- Beets
- Broccoli
- Cabbage
- Carrots
- Cauliflower
- Celery
- Corn
- Cucumbers
- Lettuce/Greens
- Mushrooms
- Onions
- Peas
- Peppers
- Potatoes
- Radishes
- Spinach
- Squash
- Sweet Potatoes
- Zucchini

## Grains

- Bagels
- Barley
- Cold Cereal
- Creamed Wheat
- Dinner Rolls
- English Muffins
- French Bread
- Hamburger Buns
- Hot Dog Buns
- Macaroni Noodles
- Oatmeal
- Pancake Mix
- Pasta Noodles
- Pita Bread
- Rice (Brown)
- Rice (White)
- Spaghetti Noodles
- Tortillas
- Whole Wheat Bread Fruits

## Fruits

- Apples
- Avocado
- Bananas
- Blackberries
- Blueberries
- Cantaloupe
- Cherries
- Cranberries
- Grapefruit
- Grapes
- Honeydew
- Kiwi
- Lemons
- Limes
- Mango
- Melon
- Nectarines
- Olives
- Oranges
- Peaches
- Pears
- Pineapple
- Plums
- Raspberries
- Stawberries
- Tomatoes
- Watermelon

## Nuts & Seeds

- Almonds
- Brazil Nuts
- Cashews
- Flaxseed
- Hazelnuts
- Macadamia
- Peanuts
- Pecans
- Pine Nuts
- Pistachios
- Pumpkin Seeds
- Sesame Seeds
- Sunflower Seeds
- Walnuts

## Protein

### Seafood

- Catfish
- Clams
- Cod
- Crab
- Halibut
- Lobster
- Mussels
- Oysters
- Salmon
- Snapper
- Shrimp
- Tilapia
- Tuna

### Meat

- Bacon/ Sausage
- Beef
- Chicken
- Eggs
- Ham/Pork
- Hot Dogs
- Lunch Meat
- Steak
- Turkey

### Legumes

- Black Beans
- Black-eyed Peas
- Garbanzo Beans
- Great Northern Beans
- Kidney Beans
- Lentils
- Lima Beans
- Pinto Beans
- Red Beans
- Small White Beans
- Soybeans
- Split Peas

# Weekly Grocery List

## Dairy
- ☐ Butter/Margarine
- ☐ Cream Cheese
- ☐ Milk
- ☐ Sour Cream
- ☐ Whipped Cream
- ☐ Yogurt

## Cheese
- ☐ Bleu Cheese
- ☐ Cheddar
- ☐ Cottage Cheese
- ☐ Cream Cheese
- ☐ Feta
- ☐ Goat Cheese
- ☐ Mozzarella
- ☐ Muenster
- ☐ Parmesan
- ☐ Provolone
- ☐ Ricotta
- ☐ Swiss

## Baking/ Dry
- ☐ Baking Powder
- ☐ Baking Soda
- ☐ Bread Crumbs
- ☐ Cornmeal
- ☐ Cornstarch
- ☐ Flour
- ☐ Sugar (Brown)
- ☐ Sugar (Powder)
- ☐ Sugar (White)
- ☐ Vanilla
- ☐ Yeast

## Weight loss Helps
- ☐ Gum
- ☐ Hard Candies/Mints
- ☐ Waterbottle
- ☐ Zero Calorie Drinks

## Healthy Snacks
- ☐ Dried Fruit
- ☐ Graham Crackers
- ☐ Granola Bars
- ☐ Popcorn
- ☐ Pretzels

## Sauces/Oils
- ☐ Canola Oil
- ☐ Hot Sauce
- ☐ Olive Oil
- ☐ Soy Sauce
- ☐ Spaghetti Sauce
- ☐ Syrup
- ☐ Vegetable Oil
- ☐ Vinegar

## Canned Foods
- ☐ Applesauce
- ☐ Beans
- ☐ Broth
- ☐ Chili
- ☐ Fruits
- ☐ Soup
- ☐ Tomato Sauce

*Notes:*

## Spices & Herbs
- ☐ Basil
- ☐ Black Pepper
- ☐ Cilantro
- ☐ Cinnamon
- ☐ Garlic
- ☐ Ginger
- ☐ Mint
- ☐ Oregano
- ☐ Paprika
- ☐ Parsley
- ☐ Red Pepper
- ☐ Salt

## Condiments
- ☐ BBQ Sauce
- ☐ Croutons
- ☐ Honey
- ☐ Jam/Jelly
- ☐ Ketchup
- ☐ Mayonnaise
- ☐ Mustard
- ☐ Peanut Butter
- ☐ Pickles
- ☐ Salad Dressing
- ☐ Salsa

# Weekly Grocery List

## Vegetables

- ☐ Asparagus
- ☐ Beets
- ☐ Broccoli
- ☐ Cabbage
- ☐ Carrots
- ☐ Cauliflower
- ☐ Celery
- ☐ Corn
- ☐ Cucumbers
- ☐ Lettuce/Greens
- ☐ Mushrooms
- ☐ Onions
- ☐ Peas
- ☐ Peppers
- ☐ Potatoes
- ☐ Radishes
- ☐ Spinach
- ☐ Squash
- ☐ Sweet Potatoes
- ☐ Zucchini

## Grains

- ☐ Bagels
- ☐ Barley
- ☐ Cold Cereal
- ☐ Creamed Wheat
- ☐ Dinner Rolls
- ☐ English Muffins
- ☐ French Bread
- ☐ Hamburger Buns
- ☐ Hot Dog Buns
- ☐ Macaroni Noodles
- ☐ Oatmeal
- ☐ Pancake Mix
- ☐ Pasta Noodles
- ☐ Pita Bread
- ☐ Rice (Brown)
- ☐ Rice (White)
- ☐ Spaghetti Noodles
- ☐ Tortillas
- ☐ Whole Wheat Bread Fruits

## Fruits

- ☐ Apples
- ☐ Avocado
- ☐ Bananas
- ☐ Blackberries
- ☐ Blueberries
- ☐ Cantaloupe
- ☐ Cherries
- ☐ Cranberries
- ☐ Grapefruit
- ☐ Grapes
- ☐ Honeydew
- ☐ Kiwi
- ☐ Lemons
- ☐ Limes
- ☐ Mango
- ☐ Melon
- ☐ Nectarines
- ☐ Olives
- ☐ Oranges
- ☐ Peaches
- ☐ Pears
- ☐ Pineapple
- ☐ Plums
- ☐ Raspberries
- ☐ Stawberries
- ☐ Tomatoes
- ☐ Watermelon

## Nuts & Seeds

- ☐ Almonds
- ☐ Brazil Nuts
- ☐ Cashews
- ☐ Flaxseed
- ☐ Hazelnuts
- ☐ Macadamia
- ☐ Peanuts
- ☐ Pecans
- ☐ Pine Nuts
- ☐ Pistachios
- ☐ Pumpkin Seeds
- ☐ Sesame Seeds
- ☐ Sunflower Seeds
- ☐ Walnuts

## Protein

### Seafood

- ☐ Catfish
- ☐ Clams
- ☐ Cod
- ☐ Crab
- ☐ Halibut
- ☐ Lobster
- ☐ Mussels
- ☐ Oysters
- ☐ Salmon
- ☐ Snapper
- ☐ Shrimp
- ☐ Tilapia
- ☐ Tuna

### Meat

- ☐ Bacon/ Sausage
- ☐ Beef
- ☐ Chicken
- ☐ Eggs
- ☐ Ham/Pork
- ☐ Hot Dogs
- ☐ Lunch Meat
- ☐ Steak
- ☐ Turkey

### Legumes

- ☐ Black Beans
- ☐ Black-eyed Peas
- ☐ Garbanzo Beans
- ☐ Great Northern Beans
- ☐ Kidney Beans
- ☐ Lentils
- ☐ Lima Beans
- ☐ Pinto Beans
- ☐ Red Beans
- ☐ Small White Beans
- ☐ Soybeans
- ☐ Split Peas

# Weekly Grocery List

## Dairy
- ☐ Butter/Margarine
- ☐ Cream Cheese
- ☐ Milk
- ☐ Sour Cream
- ☐ Whipped Cream
- ☐ Yogurt

## Cheese
- ☐ Bleu Cheese
- ☐ Cheddar
- ☐ Cottage Cheese
- ☐ Cream Cheese
- ☐ Feta
- ☐ Goat Cheese
- ☐ Mozzarella
- ☐ Muenster
- ☐ Parmesan
- ☐ Provolone
- ☐ Ricotta
- ☐ Swiss

## Baking/ Dry
- ☐ Baking Powder
- ☐ Baking Soda
- ☐ Bread Crumbs
- ☐ Cornmeal
- ☐ Cornstarch
- ☐ Flour
- ☐ Sugar (Brown)
- ☐ Sugar (Powder)
- ☐ Sugar (White)
- ☐ Vanilla
- ☐ Yeast

## Weight loss Helps
- ☐ Gum
- ☐ Hard Candies/Mints
- ☐ Waterbottle
- ☐ Zero Calorie Drinks

## Healthy Snacks
- ☐ Dried Fruit
- ☐ Graham Crackers
- ☐ Granola Bars
- ☐ Popcorn
- ☐ Pretzels

## Sauces/Oils
- ☐ Canola Oil
- ☐ Hot Sauce
- ☐ Olive Oil
- ☐ Soy Sauce
- ☐ Spaghetti Sauce
- ☐ Syrup
- ☐ Vegetable Oil
- ☐ Vinegar

## Canned Foods
- ☐ Applesauce
- ☐ Beans
- ☐ Broth
- ☐ Chili
- ☐ Fruits
- ☐ Soup
- ☐ Tomato Sauce

*Notes:*

## Spices & Herbs
- ☐ Basil
- ☐ Black Pepper
- ☐ Cilantro
- ☐ Cinnamon
- ☐ Garlic
- ☐ Ginger
- ☐ Mint
- ☐ Oregano
- ☐ Paprika
- ☐ Parsley
- ☐ Red Pepper
- ☐ Salt

## Condiments
- ☐ BBQ Sauce
- ☐ Croutons
- ☐ Honey
- ☐ Jam/Jelly
- ☐ Ketchup
- ☐ Mayonnaise
- ☐ Mustard
- ☐ Peanut Butter
- ☐ Pickles
- ☐ Salad Dressing
- ☐ Salsa

## Weekly Grocery List

### Vegetables
- Asparagus
- Beets
- Broccoli
- Cabbage
- Carrots
- Cauliflower
- Celery
- Corn
- Cucumbers
- Lettuce/Greens
- Mushrooms
- Onions
- Peas
- Peppers
- Potatoes
- Radishes
- Spinach
- Squash
- Sweet Potatoes
- Zucchini

### Grains
- Bagels
- Barley
- Cold Cereal
- Creamed Wheat
- Dinner Rolls
- English Muffins
- French Bread
- Hamburger Buns
- Hot Dog Buns
- Macaroni Noodles
- Oatmeal
- Pancake Mix
- Pasta Noodles
- Pita Bread
- Rice (Brown)
- Rice (White)
- Spaghetti Noodles
- Tortillas
- Whole Wheat Bread Fruits

### Fruits
- Apples
- Avocado
- Bananas
- Blackberries
- Blueberries
- Cantaloupe
- Cherries
- Cranberries
- Grapefruit
- Grapes
- Honeydew
- Kiwi
- Lemons
- Limes
- Mango
- Melon
- Nectarines
- Olives
- Oranges
- Peaches
- Pears
- Pineapple
- Plums
- Raspberries
- Stawberries
- Tomatoes
- Watermelon

### Nuts & Seeds
- Almonds
- Brazil Nuts
- Cashews
- Flaxseed
- Hazelnuts
- Macadamia
- Peanuts
- Pecans
- Pine Nuts
- Pistachios
- Pumpkin Seeds
- Sesame Seeds
- Sunflower Seeds
- Walnuts

### Protein

#### Seafood
- Catfish
- Clams
- Cod
- Crab
- Halibut
- Lobster
- Mussels
- Oysters
- Salmon
- Snapper
- Shrimp
- Tilapia
- Tuna

#### Meat
- Bacon/ Sausage
- Beef
- Chicken
- Eggs
- Ham/Pork
- Hot Dogs
- Lunch Meat
- Steak
- Turkey

#### Legumes
- Black Beans
- Black-eyed Peas
- Garbanzo Beans
- Great Northern Beans
- Kidney Beans
- Lentils
- Lima Beans
- Pinto Beans
- Red Beans
- Small White Beans
- Soybeans
- Split Peas

# Weekly Grocery List

## Dairy
- ☐ Butter/Margarine
- ☐ Cream Cheese
- ☐ Milk
- ☐ Sour Cream
- ☐ Whipped Cream
- ☐ Yogurt

## Cheese
- ☐ Bleu Cheese
- ☐ Cheddar
- ☐ Cottage Cheese
- ☐ Cream Cheese
- ☐ Feta
- ☐ Goat Cheese
- ☐ Mozzarella
- ☐ Muenster
- ☐ Parmesan
- ☐ Provolone
- ☐ Ricotta
- ☐ Swiss

## Baking/ Dry
- ☐ Baking Powder
- ☐ Baking Soda
- ☐ Bread Crumbs
- ☐ Cornmeal
- ☐ Cornstarch
- ☐ Flour
- ☐ Sugar (Brown)
- ☐ Sugar (Powder)
- ☐ Sugar (White)
- ☐ Vanilla
- ☐ Yeast

## Weight loss Helps
- ☐ Gum
- ☐ Hard Candies/Mints
- ☐ Waterbottle
- ☐ Zero Calorie Drinks

## Healthy Snacks
- ☐ Dried Fruit
- ☐ Graham Crackers
- ☐ Granola Bars
- ☐ Popcorn
- ☐ Pretzels

## Sauces/Oils
- ☐ Canola Oil
- ☐ Hot Sauce
- ☐ Olive Oil
- ☐ Soy Sauce
- ☐ Spaghetti Sauce
- ☐ Syrup
- ☐ Vegetable Oil
- ☐ Vinegar

## Canned Foods
- ☐ Applesauce
- ☐ Beans
- ☐ Broth
- ☐ Chili
- ☐ Fruits
- ☐ Soup
- ☐ Tomato Sauce

*Notes:*

## Spices & Herbs
- ☐ Basil
- ☐ Black Pepper
- ☐ Cilantro
- ☐ Cinnamon
- ☐ Garlic
- ☐ Ginger
- ☐ Mint
- ☐ Oregano
- ☐ Paprika
- ☐ Parsley
- ☐ Red Pepper
- ☐ Salt

## Condiments
- ☐ BBQ Sauce
- ☐ Croutons
- ☐ Honey
- ☐ Jam/Jelly
- ☐ Ketchup
- ☐ Mayonnaise
- ☐ Mustard
- ☐ Peanut Butter
- ☐ Pickles
- ☐ Salad Dressing
- ☐ Salsa

## Helpful Resources

There are a multitude of resources from which you can obtain additional helpful information to assist you in your weight loss efforts and new wellness oriented lifestyle. Education and the acquisition of new knowledge and skills is not only empowering, but can be fun and exciting. Take the time to investigate and discover various online sites and other resources for information – healthy recipes, new and applicable weight loss information and exercise options, behavior modification strategies, etc. – to further build your arsenal of effective healthy life management skills. The space below is provided for you to list those sites (addresses, etc.) that you discover as you ***act*** to develop further knowledge and understanding in your season of change and becoming.

| Site/Reference | Information Topic |
|---|---|
| | |
| | |
| | |
| | |
| | |
| | |
| | |
| | |
| | |
| | |
| | |
| | |
| | |
| | |
| | |
| | |
| | |
| | |
| | |
| | |
| | |
| | |

Made in the USA
San Bernardino, CA
22 January 2015